Getting Through

Communicating When Someone You Care For Has Alzheimer's Disease

Elizabeth Ostuni

Mary Jo Santo Pietro

The Speech Bin
Vero Beach, Florida

DEDICATION

To our patients and their loved ones

©1986, 1991 by Elizabeth Ostuni and Mary Jo Santo Pietro

All rights reserved. Permission is granted for the user to reproduce pages so indicated in limited form for instructional use only. No other parts of this book may be reproduced or transmitted in any form or by any means, electronic or mechanical, including photocopying and recording, or by any information storage and retrieval system, without written permission from the publisher.

    The Speech Bin, Inc.
    1965 Twenty-Fifth Avenue
    Vero Beach, Florida 32960

ISBN 0-937857-01-7
Catalog Number 1331
Library of Congress Catalog Card Number 86-61472

Printed in the United States of America

TABLE OF CONTENTS

Foreword v

Preface vi

Introduction viii
    Communication and Alzheimer's Disease
    Making Changes

I   Your Loved One: The Person with Dementia 1
    Problems Related to Normal Aging
    Problems Related to Other Conditions
       Sensory Conditions
          Vision
          Hearing
       Physical Conditions
          Oral Hygiene
          Balance and Movement
       Medical Conditions
       Nutrition
       Grooming
       Depression
    Primary Communication Disorders Related to Normal Aging

II   You: The Caregiver 14
    Communicating with Others: What's Your Style?
    Old Habits
    Hidden Feelings That Influence Communication
    Tough Communication Situations That Caregivers Face
    Ineffective Communication Tactics
    Keeping in Touch with Yourself and the World

III   Getting Through to Each Other 25
    Improving the Bonds of Communication
       Getting and Maintaining Attention
       Making Language Work: Getting More out of Less
    Creating Success
       Using Verbal Praise
       Using the Sense of Touch
       Using People: Children, Grandchildren, Friends, and Relatives
          Shaping Attitudes: Words and Actions
          Arranging Visits

    Using Activities
      Music, Rhythm, and Exercise
      Pets
      Language Exercises
      Life Review Diary
   Dealing with Difficult Behaviors
     Prevention
     Limiting or Stopping Unpleasant Behaviors
     Involving Others: A Good Idea
   Coping with the Blind Alzheimer's Patient

IV. Getting Through Together: The Communication Environment 47
   Home
   The Nursing Home

V Communicating as a Consumer/Advocate 52
   Knowing What to Get; Getting What You Need
   Getting Through: Communicating with Your Physician
   Getting Through: Communicating with Your Attorney
   Getting Through: Communicating with Your Home Health Aide
   Getting Through: Communicating with a Nursing Home Administrator

A Final Word 72

Appendix 73
   Healthcare Professionals: Consumer Information
   Where to Get More Information

References 85

About the Authors 86

FOREWORD

In 1907 Alois Alzheimer described the disease that has since come to bear his name. His initial report emphasized the patient's difficulty with spoken language and writing and drew attention to the fact that a communication defect characteristically accompanies this illness. Despite the early concern with language and communication disturbances, many recent investigators have concentrated on the memory abnormalities and have largely ignored the interpersonal communication disturbances. Filling this gap in our understanding of Alzheimer's disease has become an urgent issue as the number of victims steadily increases. *Getting Through: Communicating When Someone You Care For Has Alzheimer's Disease* represents an important step toward helping families understand the communication difficulties of Alzheimer's disease. It is the first book to focus on this aspect of patient-caregiver interaction.

In its approach to the patient, *Getting Through* adopts a geriatric perspective emphasizing elements of normal aging – poor hearing, poor dentition, nutritional disturbances, depression, medical diseases – that can impair communication as well as those abnormalities more specifically associated with Alzheimer's disease and other dementing illnesses. Communication is considered in its broadest sense to include memory, comprehension, linguistic skills, and social communication abilities (pragmatics). Furthermore, dementia is divided into early, middle, and late phases, and suggestions for facilitating communication are tailored to each progressive stage.

The growing size of the Alzheimer's disease population has drawn national attention to this disorder. Researchers have initiated neurobiologic investigations into the causes, clinical manifestations, and potential treatments of Alzheimer's disease. In this concern to learn more about the disease itself, however, one set of victims has gone unnoticed – the families.

Getting Through accepts the challenge of developing an ecology of communication and emphasizes the roles of both patient and family member.

The authors also respond to a commonly voiced concern of families – "What can I do?" – by providing concrete realistic suggestions for how a caregiver can facilitate communication with their intellectually impaired member. Again, using the broadest approach to communication, suggestions are given that may improve many aspects of the life of the Alzheimer's patient, including the use of music and pets. Optimism is tempered by realism, and methods are presented to aid in redirecting or modifying the potentially resistive and difficult behavior of some Alzheimer's patients. Particularly difficult problems, such as teaching grandchildren about Alzheimer's disease and easing the patient's transition from living at home to living in a nursing home, are also addressed.

Finally, *Getting Through* provides Alzheimer's families with suggestions for how to communicate with the many professionals they will meet as a result of the patient's disease. Family members must act as advocates for the patient as they make difficult decisions regarding home care, diagnostic evaluation, and treatment. They must also make complex and emotionally laden decisions regarding estate management, conservatorship, nursing home placement, and autopsy. Practical advice regarding each of these issues is provided.

Alzheimer's disease is currently the fourth leading cause of death in the United States. Dementia victims occupy more than half of all nursing home beds in this country, and more than twenty billion dollars are spent annually on the care of dementia patients. Already staggering, the burden on families and health care resources is bound to increase as the number of Alzheimer's patients increases. *Getting Through,* with its practical humanism and optimistic realism, provides guidelines that will aid caregivers, friends, relatives, and professionals as they strive to meet the challenge posed by this tragic disorder.

JEFFREY L. CUMMINGS, M.D.
Director, Neurobehavior Unit
Assistant Professor of Neurology in Residence
UCLA School of Medicine
April 14, 1986

PREFACE

Our primary purpose in writing *Getting Through: Communicating When Someone You Care For Has Alzheimer's Disease* was to develop a useful tool for those of you who have a family member or friend with Alzheimer's disease or related disorder. At every turn of this difficult road, you may find that attempts at communication – the most casual statement, well-intentioned offer, or sincere request – can have disastrous results. A once mild-mannered mate is now constantly cantankerous; a sister with whom you were close has become suspicious and negative; your mother can no longer follow the simplest of directions. In short, communication seems impossible.

Our goals are to help you discover occasions when effective communication does occur though you may not realize it; to point out some times when improved communication is a possibility; and to suggest a variety of ways to bring about that improvement.

Those of you with primary responsibility for your relative or loved one are also coming into contact with a whole new set of professionals. You are discussing symptoms, behaviors, and plans with which you may have had little prior experience. To help you in these unfamiliar situations, we have developed several sets of questions. The questions have been grouped according to the professional person with whom you will be speaking: physician, attorney, home health aide, or nursing home administrator. By using these questions, you can more easily take notes during your conversations and later recall what was discussed.

We have found the primary caregivers are not the only people who need strategies for better communication. In our aging society most of us have a dear friend, business associate, or relative who has Alzheimer's or a related disease. *Getting Through* is also for that wider circle of acquaintances who, quite naturally, look upon visits to their stricken friends or relatives with a sense of awkwardness, guilt, or distaste. What to say? What to do? How to react? Whether you are a friend, relative, or member of a volunteer outreach group, we hope our explanations and suggestions for communicating with the demented person will be of benefit to you.

Finally, it was our intention to provide a reference for individuals working in the healthcare fields. Healthcare personnel also need to become better informed about how to recognize and respond to the communicative patterns of the person with dementia. Healthcare personnel have a responsibility to look for clues in the patient's "gibberish," to adopt the role of sensitive interpreter, and to provide instruction and conversation that have the best chance of being understood. Recognizing the value of human communication is any important aspect of quality patient care.

Service providers, such as social workers, family counselors, clergy, and lawyers, should be alert to the symptomatology of communication disorders in dementia and the strategies for dealing with the problems it presents. Individuals in the helping professions may also find the chapter on communication between caregivers and professionals useful.

The title we chose, *Getting Through: Communicating When Someone You Care For Has Alzheimer's Disease,* is not directed exclusively to communication problems in Alzheimer's disease. Although Alzheimer's is the most common, there are several conditions, such as multi-infarct dementia, Huntingtons, or Creutsfeld-Jakob, that can cause what used to be called "senile dementia" or simply "senility."

Communication problems do vary from one type of dementia to another. However, some *similar* communication patterns can be identified across all dementias. Similar problems suggest similar approaches in management. Therefore, even if the diagnosis of dementia is not specifically Alzheimer's, this workbook is recommended to individuals who care for persons with any dementing illness. When we refer to people with Alzheimer's disease, we are also addressing the problems of individuals with related disorders.

When writing any book, it is important, but difficult, to come to terms with equitable references to the sexes. We have chosen to alternate between male and female references rather than use the awkward and cumbersome "he/she." We trust that our chosen convention will result in easy reading for you.

Finally, we gratefully acknowledge the persons

who assisted in the development and completion of this book:

To Marilyn Richards, Alzheimer's family member; Family Counselor to Alzheimer's families; lecturer and consultant in Alzheimer's disease: for her generous contribution of time and advice on "Communicating with a Nursing Home Administrator."

To Gary Mazart, Esq., Senior Assistant, Strauss and Wolf Law Firm, with offices in New York and New Jersey; and consultant to families on behalf of the institutionalized elderly: for his guidance in designing a questionnaire for families needing legal advice and information in "Communicating with Your Lawyer."

To Richard Mayeux, M.D., Associate Professor of Clinical Neurology and Psychiatry, Columbia College of Surgeons, and Director of the Alzheimer's Disease Research Group at columbia Presbyterian Medical Center, New York City: for his insightful recommendations for families in the section about "Communicating with Your Physician."

To Maura Coleman, M.S.W., Director of Special Programs, Visiting Homemaker Service of Morris County, Morris Plains, New Jersey: for sharing her extensive knowledge on families in need of help on "Communicating with Your Home Health Aide."

To Lynn J. Holland, Ph.D., Consultant in Gerontology at Family Life Services, Belle Fourche, and Staff Speech-Language Pathologist at Fort Meade, South Dakota, Veterans Administration Hospital: for her kind permission to adapt and recommend the *Life Review Diary* for use with the Alzheimer's patient.

To Sidney Pitts: for his patience and skill in typing and coordinating the manuscript.

To those healthcare professionals who took the time to provide us with specific information about the credentials, settings, and services that are available to both normal and impaired aging persons:

Judy Amir, M.S.W.
Linda Fein, M.S.N, R.N.C.
Ann Anderson, M.S, CCC-A
Shan Li Chen, M.B.A., R.D.
Rosemarie Bernick, R.N., M.S.N.
Ruth Manzo, O.T.R.
Maura Coleman, M.S.W.
Billie Jean O'Brien, R.N., M.S.N.
Ellen DeCotiis, M.S., CCC-SLP
Mary Lou Schmurr, R.A.
John Diffley, R.P.T.
Girija Sundar, M.A., CCC-A

And to those many interested and dedicated souls who read our manuscript, providing us with support and constructive critical feedback: you have our sincerest thanks and appreciation.

ELIZABETH OSTUNI, M.A.
MARY JO SANTO PIETRO, Ph.D.

INTRODUCTION

Communication and Alzheimer's Disease

If you are reading this book, you have probably recently received some of the most difficult news imaginable: Someone you care for has Alzheimer's disease or dementia. If your loved one is typical of the two to four million cases in the United States today (Cross and Gurland, 1985), this diagnosis was made after months of watching your loved one fail in small ways. You may have spent weeks going from specialist to specialist looking for an explanation for lapses in memory, days of depression, and moments of poor judgment.

You have probably also discovered that one of the biggest problems you face in coping with this disease is communicating with the loved one who is afflicted. The communication that used to be such a simple and automatic process between you is now difficult and labored, if not impossible. When Marian Roach, author of *Another Name for Madness,* was asked on the *Today Show* what was the worst thing about having a mother with Alzheimer's disease, she answered without hesitation, "The loss of communication."

Verbal communication is, after all, the ability that is uniquely human. In the most basic sense, verbal communication helps in forming perceptions of the world and making associations, judgments, and predictions. It assists in the ordering of history and environment. In a more complex way, it encourages the establishment and enrichment of our relationships with other human beings. It brings comfort and inspiration and enables individuals to achieve lifelong personal and interactive goals. As Lynn J. Holland (1984), speech-language pathologist and consultant in gerontology, has said, communication

> "...permits us to express ourselves to others, and encourages others to reveal themselves to us. It allows us to receive and transmit beyond our individual lifespans, bequeathing to the unborn what we have recalled from the past. For the elderly, communication may achieve a further, perhaps final, purpose: acknowledging, affirming and appreciating one's own life while coming to terms with death." (page 3)

Communication is "the exchange of information between two people." It is never really simple nor entirely automatic, of course. Truly effective communication places several demands on the communicators. The participants must share the same language, whether spoken, written, or nonverbal. They need a common experience, a shared vocabulary. There should be a certain respect between the speakers; each participant sends messages with the expectation of a response. Each must have the ability to perceive accurately all the cues transmitted – auditory, visual, and linguistic.

Furthermore, participants must be able to maintain attention. They should be open to each other's message and must desire to receive it. They must have an intellectual understanding of the information being transmitted. They also need sufficient short-term memory to retain each other's messages long enough to respond to them. Effective communication is goal-oriented. Effective communication is *Getting Through*.

Even in the early stages the person with Alzheimer's disease clearly lacks several of these prerequisites for effective communication. The person with dementia still seems to speak the same language. His intonation and grammar appear intact, but suddenly his experience has become limited. His world is reduced; he has less to talk about. His vocabulary appears diminished. Remembering and saying the names of things becomes difficult for him. Auditory and visual perception may be impaired. Although his reading aloud may appear unchanged, he does not seem to understand what he reads. He may miss subtle facial and gestural cues. He cannot maintain his attention for very long. Depression can interfere, and curiosity seems strangely absent. Humor and sarcasm are lost on him.

Often the person knows *something* is happening to him, and with that knowledge comes fear. Frightened, he tries to conceal his shortcomings by avoiding the challenge of interpersonal communication. He dismisses conversations as trivial, or he simply refuses to engage in them. Of course, what is really happening is that he does not understand the conversation and finds it easier not to participate.

When he initiates a conversation, he may repeat himself over and over, forgetting what he has already said. He may rattle on endlessly about a single thought or idea. The combination of his fear and loss of inhibitory mechanisms may also cause him to use abusive language that embarrasses the listener. Effective communication is extremely difficult. He is not *Getting Through*.

As the disease progresses, the mechanics of speech may continue to seem surprisingly intact, but the patient may become increasingly apathetic towards others and the environment. His language becomes self-centered; repetition of ideas is more and more common. He substitutes terms like "thing" and "that one" for substantive meaningful nouns. His conversation is vague, empty, and often irrelevant. He no longer seems to be able to string ideas together. He can no longer adequately manage a sequence of household chores, financial arrangements, or medications.

However, it is quite possible that not all of the communication problems your companion is experiencing stem from Alzheimer's disease. Some come from changes in life style; others may come from physical and psychological changes.

The person for whom you are caring is undoubtedly going through many overwhelming changes. He is becoming confined to his home but no longer able to be in charge of it. His daily environment and routines have changed dramatically; so have the number and types of people with whom he comes in contact. The kinds of things he has to say and the people to whom he says them are different. The ways in which other people communicate with him may have changed as well.

Your companion is also likely to be undergoing several physical changes independent of the dementing condition. For example, nearly half of people over 55 experience hearing loss that makes understanding conversation difficult and causes them to talk too loudly. Dental problems may cause speech to sound garbled or slushy. Medication can interfere with alertness, language formulation, or clear diction. Depression may make the Alzheimer's victim seem apathetic or disoriented. Any of these factors may combine with Alzheimer's in a snowballing effect that produces a dramatic and perhaps sudden decline in communicative effectiveness. These factors will be discussed in detail in the chapters that follow.

To summarize, communicating with the person you care for becomes increasingly difficult, for many reasons, at a time when the need to communicate may be more important than ever before. When individuals become older and increasingly dependent, they must rely heavily on effective communication with others to meet their needs. As you assume the role of caregiver to an Alzheimer's patient, you are facing the double-bind situation of helping a very needy person who has very severe communication problems.

Can these communication problems be totally eliminated? No, they cannot.

Although medical science has made many promising discoveries in recent years, nothing has yet been found that will stop or reverse the course of Alzheimer's disease. The painful decline of your loved one is inevitable, and his communication difficulties will persist.

Can the present communication interactions between you and the Alzheimer's patient become more effective? Yes, they can. Absolutely.

Our work and the research of many others has shown us that there are many steps caregivers can take which are likely to result in more effective communication interactions with Alzheimer's patients. This book describes a number of techniques you can use to reduce the silent space that may have grown between you and your loved one.

Can the inevitable decline of Alzheimer's disease be slowed? Recent research tells us, "Yes, it can. To some extent."

Evidence exists which indicates that patients with good physical health who remain in their homes or in the homes of loved ones, maintaining optimum communication with both caregivers and the outside world, decline less rapidly. It appears that when patients make maximum use of their remaining abilities, they maintain those abilities longer (Rowe and Besdine, 1982).

So what *can* be changed? What can be done to make communication more effective and slow the decline? In the following chapters you will find suggestions to help you enhance and maintain vital communication with your failing loved one.

Making Changes

Communication between you and your loved one with Alzheimer's can be thought of as a model with four essential components:

- the person with dementia;
- the caregiver;
- the communication between caregiver and patients; and
- the communication environment.

Definite changes can and must be made in *all four* of these components if communication is to be improved and maintained for as long as possible. This workbook is designed to help you, the caregiver

- understand the nature and importance of each of these components;
- identify the changes that must be made to improve the communication;
- make those changes successfully; and,
- establish successful communication with "outsiders": family, friends, professionals, and others.

Chapter One

THE PERSON WITH DEMENTIA

In this chapter the person with dementia will be discussed as one, but only one, of the four major components in the communication model. The nature of the problems she brings to the communication process because of normal age-related life changes, deficits due to other unrelated physical and psychological disorders, and finally as a direct result of the dementia itself will be described.

Problems Related to "Normal Aging"

The typical patient with Alzheimer's disease is at least fifty years old. She therefore brings to the communication process all the stresses that may come with normal aging. Growing older introduces an assortment of physical, social, and psychological problems for which most people are not well prepared. A primary experience of aging is the experience of loss: Loss of family and friends due to life changes and death; loss of health; loss of livelihood, social role, and physical attractiveness; and loss of independence, both financial and physical. The faculties of eyesight, hearing, touch, smell, and taste may diminish as well. Under the best of circumstances adjustment to these changes can be difficult.

In caring for an aging Alzheimer's patient, you will find communication affected by these common losses in many ways. Chances are, many people with whom she once communicated may now be living in warmer climates or deceased. Others may no longer visit to save you, or themselves, embarrassment. Perhaps her children live at a distance. Her spouse also may have died. So beyond the pain of loss, there is the very real question of with whom does she communicate.

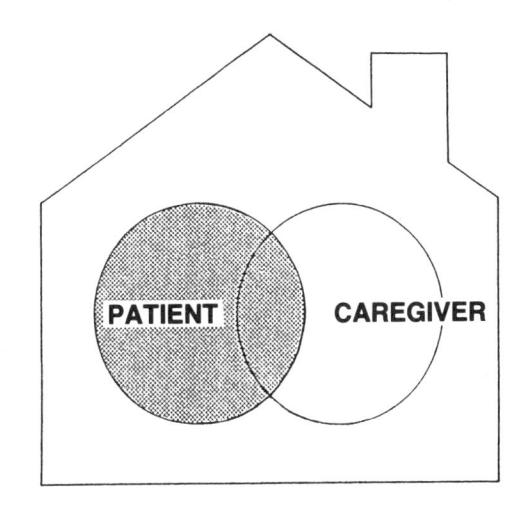

If she is over 65, she is probably also coping with one or more additional medical conditions. The average American over 65 has 3.6 "important disabilities," such as diabetes, hearing problems, or high blood pressure (Rowe and Besdine, 1982). Stated simply, communication with others is always more difficult when one does not feel well.

Remember that once people have retired, whether their jobs involved executive management, truck driving, or child rearing, one of their major repertoires of communicative interactions is lost. A whole familiar vocabulary of job-related words may no longer be needed. The casual communication partners of the workplace are no longer available. There can be a feeling of isolation, real or imagined. Worse, some people may struggle with a perceived loss of identity and find it difficult to know exactly how to relate to others. Retired persons may wonder, "What do people expect me to say now that I don't work as a doctor, a teacher, a foreman?" Those who no longer have a work-related identity in society or who feel that their physical attractiveness is declining may even wonder whether anyone would want to hear what they have to say.

Loss of financial independence reduces the trips, recreation, and even long distance telephone calls that can relieve the older person's isolation. Financial dependence on others often blocks open communication between relatives because it introduces new tensions. Loss of physical independence requires a whole new set of words and ways of doing things to maintain the activities of daily life.

Many older people feel, and rightly so, that they are at the mercy of their "helpers," whether these helpers are family members, neighbors, therapists, volunteer services, frozen dinners, wheelchairs, or laxatives. When a person has lost independence, it is often difficult to communicate with others on an equal plane. Sometimes younger people and persons in the helping professions treat the disabled elderly as if they were children: "Let's not be stubborn now." "It's time to take our medicine." "That's a good girl." This kind of "conversation" hardly inspires a warm reply. Besides, much if not all, of the patient's energy may now be absorbed by the basic tasks of everyday function and health.

Besides these life changes, the essential instruments for communication – hearing, vision, and touch – may also begin to weaken. Even in the best of health, an elderly person must concentrate harder to be effective at communicating because of these factors. For example, to be completely successful in the televised 1984 presidential campaign debates, President Ronald Reagan had to be sure that his opponent spoke to his ear with the hearing aid, his notes were in large print under bright light, and he could see his opponent's face clearly on a large TV monitor placed nearby.

In short, successful communication grows more difficult simply as a result of aging, even without the addition of serious illness and/or Alzheimer's disease.

Problems Related to Other Conditions

In this section the concept of *excess disability* is introduced. *Excess disability* means that the person may be suffering from a far greater handicap than is necessary because of other unrelated physical, sensory, or medical conditions that he has besides Alzheimer's disease. Someone with an excess disability in communication will have more difficulty listening, understanding, or talking if other health factors are interfering. Certainly, your friend or relative will feel more like communicating the better he feels.

The problems can occur because of normal aging or because of another illness. Such problems may seem trivial compared to the toll the dementia itself is taking on the person. You might even be tempted to think, "Why bother?", especially if treatment is expensive or inconvenient.

Make no mistake. Do not ignore these deficits because they take their toll, draining both you and the patient of much-needed energy reserves. To ignore these conditions is to invite a host of other safety and health risks. In many cases, good preventive care of these other conditions actually slows the overall process of deterioration.

The following conditions are among those that can impose an unnecessary burden on someone already suffering from dementia.

Sensory Conditions
Vision

Visual perceptual problems do sometimes occur directly as a result of Alzheimer's disease. Objects and persons may look different in shape, color, or texture. They may appear to be in a different place, to the right or left of the actual location. However, it cannot be assumed that bumping into objects or missing what is reached for is only a function of the disease. The possibility that eyesight – visual acuity – could be failing must first be considered. In addition, an eye examination will also detect other conditions, such as cataracts or glaucoma, that can interfere with the patient's well-being.

Whether the person wore glasses before the onset of Alzheimer's, his eyes should be checked while he is still able to answer the questions of the eye doctor (optometrist or ophthalmologist) with some accuracy. Both the eye physician and your relative will need your help. The eye examination room may be dark for part of the time, and your relative will not be able to see the examiner's face clearly when he speaks. These are the worst possible conditions under which to ask someone with Alzheimer's disease to respond. To assist in the eye exam, let the physician know that your relative understands questions or statements better when they are phrased in a certain way. Acting as an interpreter, repeat or rephrase questions as necessary. By all means, when you make an appointment for any examination, let the doctor's office know beforehand that you will be bringing in a special patient. The receptionist may want to schedule a slightly longer appointment time so that no one feels rushed.

The eye doctor will recommend whether glasses are needed. Even if the person you care for no longer reads, glasses can still be important for moving about safely and recognizing others. If glasses are worn, make sure they are clean and fit comfortably on the head. If he resists wearing them, check to determine if the lenses have become scratched or cloudy or the frames bent.

Hearing

Studies show that at least half of Americans over 65 have significant hearing losses. Recent research indicates that the incidence of hearing loss among persons with dementia of the Alzheimer's type is at least 20% higher than the incidence among normal elderly persons. Furthermore, hearing losses in patients with dementia tend to be more severe. Scientists are beginning to suspect that a relationship may exist between Alzheimer's disease and hearing loss (Weinstein, 1991).

Impaired hearing is a more serious problem than many people realize. There is a saying, "Blindness separates man from things, but deafness separates man from man." Even a "normal" person will gradually withdraw and become suspicious and depressed if suffering from an unidentified, untreated hearing loss. Trying to listen and understand is exhausting when hearing is poor. For the person with a dementia who is struggling with so many other problems, hearing loss is an especially serious handicap.

Many conditions contribute to the loss of hearing in our industrialized society. Hearing acuity is lost as a result of nerve damage that results from exposure to loud noise on the job, during wartime, or from recreational noise coming from machinery, hunting, or even loud music. Nerve (also known as *sensorineural*) losses can also result from high fevers or the use of certain medications. Many ear infections early in life may leave one vulnerable to later hearing loss.

Hearing acuity may also be dulled by current physical conditions that can produce *conductive* hearing losses, losses that are not the result of nerve damage. Allergies, "swimmer's ear," and fluid or wax build-up in the outer or middle ears lead to mild but annoying hearing losses. Your family physician or an otolaryngologist (ear-nose-throat specialist) may be able to prescribe medication for these conditions that can relieve "fuzzy" hearing and uncomfortable pressure in the ear.

If your loved one is going to undergo any type of clinical evaluation, it is a good idea to have his hearing examined first by an audiologist* (*see Appendix) before other testing. If a hearing loss is detected, further testing of memory, language comprehension, and related abilities should be conducted with amplification. This will insure that results of mental tests will be accurate and not made worse by an interfering hearing loss. If examiners know that a person has a hearing loss, they can also make use of appropriate lighting, face-to-face communication techniques, and a slower rate of speech to guarantee that he understands what is being said to him.

A hearing aid can provide significant help for nearly every hearing loss; however, not every Alzheimer's patient is a good candidate for a hearing aid. There are a number of factors that must be considered to determine whether a particular Alzheimer's patient is likely to be helped by wearing a hearing aid. A list of these factors was complied in 1985 by the Alzheimer's Functional Assessment Team at

**Alzheimer's Functional Assessment Team
Guidelines for Recommendation of a Hearing Aid**

1. Stage of disease, functional level of patient, and ability to cope with impairments related directly to the disease

2. Presence of other sensory, physical, or medical deficits

3. Type and severity of hearing impairment

4. Behavioral observations of the patient's tolerance for

    a. a device in the ear such as a hearing aid or other type of assistive listening device

    b. someone else assisting in placement, adjustment, and care of the aid

5. Ability and willingness of family member or primary caregiver to take responsibility for care and maintenance of the aid

6. A written agreement between family and hearing aid dispenser regarding a trial period of use (usually between 30 and 60 days) OR family member agreement to take out a special insurance policy on the aid to cover the trial period of adjustment

---

Table 1. Criteria for Decision to Recommend a Hearing Aid to the Patient with a Dementing Illness: Dover General Hospital and Medical Center, Dover, New Jersey.

Dover General Hospital in Dover, New Jersey. It appears in Table 1 on page 4. Of the criteria listed, two are probably most indicative of future success with a hearing aid. One is the willingness of the patient to tolerate the device in his ear, and the other is the willingness of a caregiver to take responsibility for the care and maintenance of the aid.

If you and the audiologist agree that your loved one might benefit from a hearing aid, one can purchased directly from an audiologist who dispenses hearing aids or from a qualified hearing aid dealer. Like eyeglasses, a hearing aid must be carefully fitted to the patient's ear and hearing ability. Usually Medicare will pay for a hearing evaluation but not for the hearing aid itself. Many insurance companies do pay for prescribed hearing aids; some agencies charge for them on a sliding scale based on ability to pay.

Once the patient is fitted with an aid, a period of adjustment must be expected. Since the person with Alzheimer's finds new learning difficult, the aid must be introduced in a slow and cautious manner. The audiologist can help you assist your loved one learn to use the hearing aid most effectively. You may see excellent results immediately; you may see no visible results at all. The first thirty days should be considered the time for trying the aid. Most states provide for a thirty-day full-refund trial period for all hearing aids. Be sure to arrange a written contract with your hearing aid dispenser to define the trial use of the aid. A low-cost insurance policy on the aid is also a good idea. Information about such policies is available from most audiologists.

If your loved one is already wearing a hearing aid, make sure it still fits well and whether it is providing adequate amplification for his present hearing level.

Other pertinent questions about the aid: Is it clean? Is wax build-up in the earmold dampening sound? Do you know how to remove the wax from the earmold?...Are the batteries functioning? Do you know how to change them? ...Is the aid properly set into the ear? A whistling feedback will result if there is any air space in the ear canal....Is the aid turned to the proper volume setting when he is wearing it? Do you know what the proper setting is? This final question is very important because if the volume is set too low, the aid will not amplify sounds enough to be helpful. If the setting is too high, the excess noise will cause the patient discomfort and reduce his tolerance for the aid.

If, after thirty days, the patient is still not wearing his aid as much as the audiologist has recommended, ask the audiologist to check for the comfort of fit in the ear canal. Sometimes relatively minor adjustments to the earmold can make the aid more tolerable and therefore more useful.

If, after all, your loved one is not a good candidate for a personal hearing aid, he might still benefit from one or more instruments called assistive listening devices (ALDs). Assistive listening devices are either wireless (FM or infrared systems) or hard-wired devices that aid the patient in such activities as watching television, talking on the telephone, listening to speakers or plays, hearing the doorbell, and having successful one-on-one conversations. An audiologist can also help you find the assistive listening devices that will be most helpful to your relative.

Physical Conditions
Oral Hygiene

Good oral hygiene and dental care are essentials in the efforts to free the individual from a state of *excess disability*. To avoid unnecessary dental expenses, make sure that your relative continues to go for regular dental checkups and that he brushes his teeth thoroughly. Since he may forget what he is doing halfway through the brushing, check often to see that the job is completed.

Also encourage frequent mouthwash and flossing. These suggestions are not for hygiene alone. Persons who wear dentures, take medicines, or eat certain foods may have unpleasant breath odor. Habitual bad breath discourages others from closeness. You will want to be sensitive to such areas of care that will make him more pleasant to be with. As with other activities of daily living, choose the language and wording of your directions carefully to get him to accept the task without resisting it. (See Chapter Three: Improving the Bonds of Communication.)

Tooth decay or poorly fitting dentures can make a difference in how much and what type of foods the person wants to eat, and how much or how little he feels like talking. Also, if he is constantly fighting loose dentures, he may find it easier not to talk. Major weight gain or weight loss can cause dentures to shift and fit improperly. He may be spending a large portion of every day uncomfortable because his dentures slip or pinch. If he has pain from a cavity or from food lodged in the gums or sores from ill-fitting dentures, his discomfort will be worse. Recall how large even the tiniest canker sore can feel on the tip of your tongue, and you will know how important good oral hygiene and dental care are.

If the patient suddenly refuses to wear dentures, this might be his only way of telling you he is having some of these problems. Pay attention to his unspoken message so that you can find out what the problem is and how to solve it for him.

Improperly fitting dentures in combination with the person's increased inattention and poor coordination can also lead to difficulty in chewing, swallowing, or to serious choking incidents. Persons with dementing conditions tend to "pocket" food inside their gums instead of chewing and swallowing as they should. The problem then becomes one of safety as well as comfort, nutrition, and ease of communication.

Consult your dentist frequently for advice and good dental care. There are a small but growing number of dentists specializing in the care of persons with dementing conditions. Since mild sedatives are sometimes used during treatment, you will want to furnish the dentist with a complete list of other medications your relative is taking.

If eating problems persist despite attention to dentures and oral hygiene, you will also find it helpful to consult a speech-language pathologist* or a registered dietician.* Some of these professionals have had additional training and experience in helping persons with dysphagia, the medical term for swallowing problems. Feel free to ask if they are qualified to treat this worrisome problem.

Balance and Movement

Balance can be a problem in elderly persons for several reasons. Impaired hearing or vision can cause them to miss sights or sounds necessary to move comfortably in their environment. Arthritis and osteoporosis can stiffen and alter movement patterns. Neurological changes in the brain may create a bent position of the back and a characteristic shuffling gait.

Communication can be affected by movement and balance problems in a variety of ways. A person who has limited ability to move may not readily turn her body toward the speaker when her name is called. She may remain rigid instead of placing herself comfortable in a conversational circle. She may have to pay so much attention to avoiding a fall that she cannot concentrate on what someone else is saying. Without question, movement and balance problems can significantly limit a person's ability to "join in." This may be perceived by others as a lack of willingness to participate. As caregiver, you will want to learn more about these problems and ask professionals how best to deal with them. You will need to communicate what you have learned with the patient to help her compensate.

Occasionally, as assistive device such as a cane can be helpful in maintaining balance. Like the hearing aid, a cane should not be introduced after the dementia has progressed too far. You might consider supplying a cane early in the disease simply as a supportive touch when going for walks. This will accustom your relative to its use and perhaps lessen

Worksheet I

STATUS OF SENSORY AND PHYSICAL CONDITIONS

SPECIALIST NAME	PHONE	DATE OF VISIT	FINDINGS	RECOMMENDATIONS
Audiologist				
Dentist				
Ear-Nose-Throat Doctor				
Eye Doctor				
Occupational Therapist				
Physiatrist				
Physical Therapist				
Speech-Language Pathologist				
Other				

© 1986 Elizabeth Ostuni and Mary Jo Santo Pietro
This form may be reproduced for personal use only.

resistance later when she may truly need the cane.

The early nontherapeutic use of a cane needs no prescription. However, a properly adjusted cane used specifically for support and balance must be prescribed by a physician. A physiatrist (doctor of rehabilitative medicine), an orthopedist, or your family physician can prescribe one for your relative. A physical therapist* can assist you in choosing the correct type, height, and use of the cane. The physical therapist should also check any other such devices your relative is using to determine whether they are still the proper size and fit for her changing stature and physique.

If your family member is an amputee and wears an artificial limb, it is essential that its proper care and fit be maintained. If you feel awkward about assuming care of the limb or the procedures are unfamiliar to you, you may obtain proper instruction from a qualified physical therapist.

Worksheet I on page 7 has been designed for your use in recording and keeping track of the status of your relative's sensory and physical conditions. It is reproducible so you may make as many copies as you need.

Be sure to review and update the information annually or more frequently if necessary. Keep the worksheet in an easily accessible place for quick reference by all caregivers.

Medical Conditions

Medical problems drain the energy and receptiveness of your loved one. Be cautious about dismissing an ailment simply as "a sign of old age" or "just another symptom of Alzheimer's disease" about which you can do nothing anyway. Even though the individual himself may be only vaguely aware of the troublesome condition, the ramifications can be great.

Begin by systematically listing your relative's known medical conditions. Use Worksheet II on page 9. This simple exercise will raise your own awareness of what each condition is, how it makes the person feel, and taken together, how these conditions can have a cumulative impact on his system.

Some medical conditions that are commonly encountered in the elderly are diabetes, arthritis, hypertension (high blood pressure), cardiac disability, cataracts, osteoporosis, and emphysema. A growing number also have Parkinson's disease that is accompanied by specific behaviors and symptoms that are quite distinct from Alzheimer's disease and often treatable.

It is also extremely important for you to know the amounts and kinds of medications that your relative is taking and what he is being treated for and why. Interactions and additive effects from several medications can make a big difference in behavior, sense of well-being, and communication skills. Many physicians report that Alzheimer's patients react differently to certain medications that other people do.

Medical conditions and the prescribed remedies affect the ability to communicate in a number of ways. Some medications change speech from clear to "slushy" or significantly reduce energy for talking. Other medicines dry out the mouth, making it uncomfortable for the person to swallow some types of foods. Still others dull taste or sensitivity to temperature or food textures. Certain medications slow reaction time and impede rapid understanding of incoming information. This increases the time necessary to respond. Medication that is prescribed to control seizures sometimes causes gums to swell and become tender.

The balancing of effective medication between too much, too little, and what is definitely necessary is an exacting science. All medical professionals who treat your Alzheimer's patient should be given a list of the kinds and dosages of the medicines he is taking so that this delicate balance can be achieved.

Worksheet II has been prepared for you to record pertinent information about the patient's medical conditions and medications. Because of the complexity of treatment re-

Worksheet II

MEDICAL CONDITIONS AND MEDICATIONS

DATE OF VISIT	CONDITION BEING TREATED	PHYSICIAN/ SPECIALIST Name/Phone	FINDINGS	RECOMMEN- DATIONS	MEDICATION AND DOSAGE	RESULTS/ BEHAVIORAL CHANGES

© 1986 Elizabeth Ostuni and Mary Jo Santo Pietro
This form may be reproduced for personal use only.

quired in Alzheimer's disease, keeping accurate records is critical.

Review and update the information on this chart at least annually or *whenever medications are changed.* Keep copies of the chart easily accessible for quick reference by all caregivers such as the visiting nurse, homemaker/health aide, and close family members.

Nutrition

Because there are so many other urgent demands in Alzheimer's, the area of nutrition is easily overlooked. Yet there are many reasons why eating is likely to become a problem: poor memory; inattention; medications that reduce taste sensation and appetite or dry out the mouth; a confusing array of food on the plate; lack of initiative or motivation to eat; poorly fitting dentures; and physical illnesses, to name a few. Any of these factors can operate alone or in combination to create a digestive or nutritional problem. Excessive weight gain or loss can quickly occur. Improper eating habits also tend to upset the intended results of medications.

A well-balanced diet is essential for the good general health of your relative. If you need help addressing specific dietary problems your relative has, consult either a nurse clinician* whose specialty is gerontology or a registered dietician.* Typically one or two consultations are sufficient to learn about the necessary dietary steps and precautions so this should not be an item of great expense.

Grooming

Personal hygiene is one skill that a person with dementia begins to neglect early in the disease. In an effort to maintain the more basic functions, a caregiver may also have difficulty attending to details like removal of food stains on clothes, attractive hairdos, changes in underwear from minor incontinencies, or the use of makeup or a razor. Why should personal appearance be a matter of importance now? You might think, "He doesn't know the difference anyway."

But recall the concept of *excess disability,* introduced earlier. As you move about in public with your relative, you will want to reduce the stigma of dementia as much as possible. Remain sensitive to how his physical appearance influences others' perception of him and their desire to approach and interact with him.

Remember such things as clothing changes, attractive and timely haircuts, deodorant, pleasant scents, shoe repair, and manicuring needs. Fuss occasionally over makeup or jewelry. Bring him a new tie or pair of socks. Join in a shoe-shining activity. Splash on the aftershave lotion; familiar scents evoke very strong memories. They remind him in a positive way about his former self and also make him more enjoyable to be with.

Depression

Up to 44% of all elderly persons may be suffering from clinical depression (Blazer and Williams, 1980). One type may be *reactive depression* that comes in response to the many life losses mentioned earlier; the elderly person may have a lot to be depressed about. Another kind of depression may be *organic depression.* It results from a medical condition, such as malnutrition or hormonal imbalance; a particular medication or combination of medications; or withdrawal of medication.

The person with depression clearly has a significant problem in communication. Apathy and withdrawal can rapidly lead to isolation. Severe depression may have several symptoms in common with dementia, such as loss of self-care, physical complaints, disorientation, and difficulties with concentration and memory. Severe depression occasionally may even be misdiagnosed as dementia. Depression, however, differs from dementia because depression has a relatively rapid onset and the patient tends to be aware of his overwhelming sadness. An examination by a qualified geriatric specialist, neuropsychiatrist, or neuropsychologist may be required to diagnose these conditions and differentiate between them.

The patient's physician should also be consulted about repeated episodes of depression. Sometimes in the early stages of Alzheimer's, reactive depression may occur because of the person's growing awareness of his own decline. Options for dealing with reactive depression are counseling for the patient; changes in living conditions, such as stabilizing routine or making the environment safe; and tender loving care.

Organic depression, on the other hand, may be a side effect of medication or a drug interaction, and it can sometimes be relieved through medical management. Depressive behavior should not be assumed to be an inevitable symptom of dementia nor should it be assumed that depressive behavior is hopeless to treat. Sometimes medications can be prescribed to relieve such symptoms; this is done more frequently in the early stages of the disease rather than later on. These antidepressive drugs are most appropriately prescribed by a physician who is skilled in geriatric medicine.

Primary Communication Disorders

Changes in speech and language begin early in Alzheimer's disease and are subtle at first. As the disease progresses, these losses become more obvious and compensation for them more difficult. By the later stages some patients may stop talking altogether and seem unaware of being spoken to.

Language deteriorates in Alzheimer's disease as a direct result of the general deterioration of brain functioning. Which functions deteriorate and the speed and degree of deterioration may vary from patient to patient. There is, however, a similar pattern of language loss in all dementing patients. Their language begins to change as the areas of the brain that serve specific speech and language functions change. Deterioration of the centers that serve word retrieval, word recognition, reading, or writing will bring about changes in those same functions. Language also breaks down because cognitive functions of the brain, such as memory and problem solving, are also crumbling. Furthermore, all intact cognitive functioning and thought become increasingly slowed as the rate of processing and understanding information is reduced. This too directly affects language.

Losses in language and speaking ability can be roughly divided into four interrelated categories: memory, comprehension, linguistic skills, and social communication. The use of language in social communication is frequently referred to by linguists and speech-language pathologists as "pragmatics." Chart I, "Language Breakdown in Persons with Alzheimer's Disease," on pages 12-13 lists the language symptoms and behaviors expected in the "early," "middle," and "late" stages of the disease. Also presented in the chart are the basic skills that are likely to be retained at each stage.

The kinds of language losses that may occur can be predicted. Understanding what is happening and approximately when it may occur increases your chances of compensating for the deficits. Compensating for language losses helps maintain good communication for as long as possible. Many suggestions for facilitating and maintaining the best possible communication are presented in the following chapters.

As you study this chart, be aware that language differences are apparent almost from the onset of the disease. Verbal expression will continue to change and become more difficult as dementia increases. You must be prepared to adapt your communication style to match and support your loved one's need to understand and be understood.

Chart I

LANGUAGE BREAKDOWN IN PERSONS WITH ALZHEIMER'S DISEASE

	MEMORY	**COMPREHENSION**

EARLY "FOR-GETFUL" STAGES	• confused about time but not about places or persons
	• experiences mild loss of long and short-term memory that is not always apparent in everyday conversation
	• experiences some loss of recently acquired information and slowness in retrieval of information
		• has difficulty understanding:
		  —complex conversation, anecdotes, etc.
		  —rapid speech
		  —speech in noisy/distracting environment
		• unable to detect humor and sarcasm
		• follows directions that are clearly stated
		• understands written cues
		• understands facial expressions, gestures, and other nonverbal emotional cues
		• shows frustration at lack of understanding

MIDDLE STAGES	• confused about time and place but not about familiar persons or self • experiences moderate loss of long and short-term memory • cannot think of less common words or concepts and less familiar names • cannot remember 3-item lists or 3-step directions • has difficulty remembering some information immediately after it has been presented	• has trouble understanding ordinary conversation • unable to process rapid speech • has difficulty focusing and maintaining attention; is distracted by noise, multiple speakers • requires repetition of simple directions • can read mechanically but does not understand meaning of what is read • misses facial cues but retains perception of emotional meaning
LATE STAGES	• is disoriented for time, place, and person • cannot form new memories • fails to recognize family members	• fails to understand word meanings • may be unaware of being spoken to

Chart I

LANGUAGE BREAKDOWN IN PERSONS WITH ALZHEIMER'S DISEASE

	LINGUISTIC SKILLS	SOCIAL COMMUNICATION (PRAGMATICS)
EARLY "FOR-GETFUL" STAGES	<ul><li>has some problems in thinking of what to say</li><li>takes longer for all language processing, hesitates and pauses more</li><li>experiences mild naming difficulties; may use related words, such as "sugar" for "salt"</li><li>often self-corrects word errors</li><li>uses good grammar and diction</li><li>circumlocutes, talking round about a topic</li></ul>	<ul><li>digresses from topic in conversation</li><li>tends to repeat himself</li><li>may ramble on and on</li><li>relies heavily on cliches</li><li>gets along adequately in most social situations</li><li>becomes angry and argumentative easily</li></ul>
MIDDLE STAGES	<ul><li>has substantial loss of naming and word-finding abilities, especially for abstract or specific words</li><li>uses more and more empty words and "related words"</li><li>processes words into ideas more slowly</li><li>cannot relate ideas or events in order</li><li>uses some jargon or "gibberish"</li><li>may perseverate, endlessly repeating questions, words, or ideas</li><li>uses relatively good grammar and diction</li></ul>	<ul><li>makes vague, empty, irrelevant conversation with many stereotypical utterances</li><li>asks fewer questions</li><li>seldom comments or self-corrects</li><li>is excessively self-oriented</li><li>does not initiate conversation</li><li>repeats ideas over and over</li><li>withdraws from difficult social situations</li><li>can still handle some casual social situations</li></ul>
LATE STAGES	<ul><li>may repeat incessantly or echo what others say</li><li>may use poor grammar and diction</li><li>may speak only in jargon or nonsense</li><li>may be mute</li></ul>	<ul><li>is no longer aware of social interaction or expectancies</li><li>withdraws partially or completely from communication</li></ul>

Chapter Two
THE CAREGIVER

It takes two to communicate. This chapter is about the second but most important component of the four-part communication model, the caregiver. YOU.

This chapter encourages you to take total responsibility for facilitating and prolonging communication with your loved one. The reason for this is clear. Simply stated, unless *you* take the responsibility, communication will not take place. In addition, by assuming this responsibility you may make your life far easier in the months and years ahead, so it is worth your time and trouble.

You will need to make the initial effort of gathering information about yourself. Next you must be prepared to let go of any old patterns of communication (or non-communication) that may no longer be effective in order to replace them with more sensitive approaches. It may seem difficult at first, but the fact that you are reading this workbook means that you want to and can be successful.

To reiterate: You are the caregiver. You must now assume primary responsibility for effective communication with the person who has Alzheimer's disease. *He no longer can.*

Since that is the case, it is important to take a good look at yourself as a communicator just as you studied the person with dementia in Chapter One. What are your strengths as a communicator? What are your weaknesses? What are *your* needs in communicating with your loved one and with the rest of the world?

In the following sections you will have the opportunity to explore:

- your personal communication style;
- old habits of communication;
- hidden feelings that could be affecting communication with your loved one;
- tough communication situations that you as a caregiver face; and
- inefficient communication tactics that you may have developed in response to your relative's deteriorating speech and language skills.

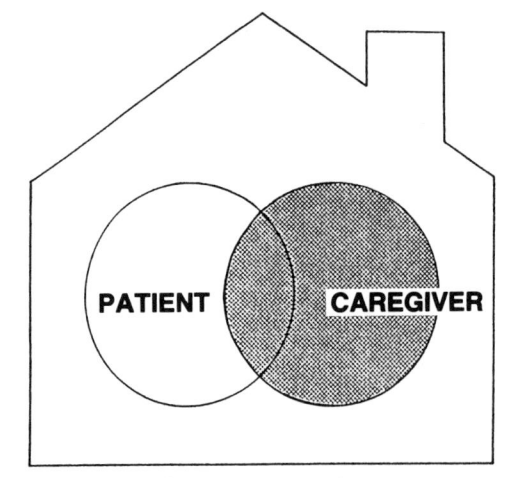

One popular method of self-assessment that has proven most successful is the questionnaire. Several such questionnaires are outlined on the following pages. Each has a slightly different design to enable you to explore most effectively the different facets of your communicative self.

Begin by reading each one through with just mild curiosity. Then write in or circle the answers requested. Finally, return to your answer sheet six months to one year from now. Have your attitudes, expectations, or communication skills changed in any way? Reexamining your answers may reveal some surprising, perhaps encouraging, information about your inner gifts and resources.

**Communicating With Others;
What's Your Style?**

First, take a look at how, when, and under what conditions you communicate most comfortably. What is your typical style of getting through to others? On pages 15-17 are 20 questions that probe your own unique way of talking and listening. Circle the number under each question that most closely describes your

Questionnaire I
COMMUNICATING WITH OTHERS; WHAT'S MY STYLE?

BEFORE I BEGAN CARING FOR AN ALZHEIMER'S PATIENT:

A. I considered myself
   1. a recluse
   2. shy
   3. an average communicator
   4. a better-than-average communicator
   5. a "real talker"

B. The amount of time a day I liked to spend interacting with others was about
   1. less than 10 minutes
   2. 10-30 minutes
   3. at least one hour
   4. generally 1-3 hours
   5. 3+ hours

C. The number of people I talked to for more than one minute on an average day was
   1. two or fewer
   2. three
   3. four or five
   4. six or seven
   5. eight or more

D. The number of phone conversations I had in a day was
   1. two or fewer
   2. three
   3. four
   4. five
   5. six or more

E. The average number of hours I spent outside the home each day was
   1. less than one
   2. one
   3. two or three
   4. three to six
   5. six or more

F. I liked my home environment to be
   1. quiet all the time
   2. quiet interrupted by occasional conversation
   3. generally quiet, but sometimes filled with people and music
   4. generally alive with people and noise but with regular quiet periods
   5. full of people, activity, and music as much as possible

G. The number of "personal" conversations, as opposed to business or social conversations, that I had on an average day was
   1. none
   2. one
   3. two
   4. three
   5. four or more

H. I wrote letters, memos, a diary
   1. never
   2. rarely
   3. occasionally; 2-4 per week
   4. frequently; approximately one a day
   5. very frequently; several a day

IN GENERAL:

I. People tell me that my rate of speech is
   1. very slow
   2. deliberate
   3. average
   4. relatively rapid
   5. too fast

J. People tell me
   1. I talk too softly
   2. I sometimes cannot be heard
   3. very little about how loud my speech is; it must be normal
   4. I sometimes talk too loudly
   5. I constantly speak in a loud voice

K. People tell me
   1. they can't understand my speech

2. I frequently mumble
3. very little about my voice and diction; it must be normal
4. my voice and diction are excellent
5. I should have been an actor!

L. I would rate my vocabulary as
1. limited
2. adequate for daily needs
3. average for American high school graduate
4. sophisticated; college graduate level
5. truly erudite

M. My use of body language is
1. minimal; I talk with my mouth only
2. infrequent; I sometimes gesture
3. frequent but limited; I gesture primarily with my hands
4. flourishing; I use everything at my disposal to get my message across
5. ample; I use gesture and touch often to make a point

N. The acuteness of my hearing
1. sometimes seems to be a problem, but I've never had it checked
2. has been checked; I could use a hearing aid but do not wear one;
3. is unknown to me
4. has been checked; is adequate (with or without an aid)
5. is excellent; I never miss a thing

O. My use of humor and sarcasm is
1. rare; people tell me I have no sense of humor
2. latent; I enjoy humor, but I can't tell a joke
3. occasional; I rely upon it once in a while
4. well-developed; I have a good sense of humor and sometimes use sarcasm
5. constant; I am known for my sense of humor and sarcastic remarks

P. I maintain eye contact during conversation
1. rarely; I seldom look at anyone
2. with difficulty; especially with authority figures and/or Alzheimer's patient
3. most of the time with friends, but not with authority figures and/or patient
4. fairly easily and fairly often with most people I encounter
5. all the time: I enjoy "staring people down"

Q. I touch a person when I communicate
1. seldom
2. occasionally with my children or mate
3. sometimes, if I know a person well
4. often when it seems appropriate to get a message across
5. frequently; I consider it a primary means of communication

R. I feel responsible for starting a conversation or introducing a new topic of conversation
1. seldom, if ever
2. occasionally
3. about half the time
4. more often than not
5. always, or so it seems to me

S. As a listener, I
1. am primarily a "good ear" and not a talker
2. prefer to listen, but talk if I have to
3. enjoy listening and responding to what I hear
4. prefer to talk, but listen if I have to
5. "am primarily a talker; I get impatient if I have to listen too long"

T. Before the person I care for developed Alzheimer's disease, we communicated with each other
1. very little; less than one contact per day
2. daily, in superficial conversation
3. frequently in everyday conversations
4. daily, providing each other with some emotional support
5. daily, with frequent intimate conversations providing strong emotional support

Questionnaire I
COMMUNICATING WITH OTHERS; WHAT'S MY STYLE?

SCORE

Below 20	Very introverted communication style; taking primary responsibility for communication with the patient or as a consumer/advocate will be difficult
40-59	Primarily a listener; may need encouragement to take initiative; should be able to adapt communication style effectively for the roles of caregiver and advocacy
60-79	Outgoing talker; may need to practice listening skills; should be good advocate with healthcare professionals
80-100	Very extroverted communication style; may have difficulty modifying habits to encourage communication with Alzheimer's patients

IMPORTANT! Do not place a value judgment on your personal style of communication. Rather, be aware of the characteristics of your communication style so that you can adapt it for more effective interaction with the Alzheimer's patient and the outside world.

communication style then total all the numbers. The scale at the end of the questionnaire suggests what your total score means in meeting the communication needs of someone with dementia.

Old Habits

Success in adapting your personal communication style to your new circumstances depends heavily on the old communication habits you and the patient have developed together over the years. Whether you had an extremely intimate relationship or a distant one, you will now need to adjust to changing communication needs.

For example, in some marriages, the husband consistently acts in the role of breadwinner and "boss." He expects to assume the leading role in conversation and decision-making. When Alzheimer's disease limits his ability to play that role, he becomes frustrated and angry. When his wife must take over the responsibility for communication and decision-making, she is often overwhelmed and may be resentful. Conversely, the woman who has always been in charge of her own home may deal very badly with being "mothered" by those she cared for so many years. Some couples have communicated on only a surface level for years. Others have relationships that thrive on cutting words and juicy arguments. Some parent-child relationships are filled with old resentments, never to be resolved now that the parent has Alzheimer's disease.

Some parents are uncomfortable being parented by their children, while many grown children find it nearly impossible to reverse roles and tell their parents what to do, Sometimes a close friend feels truly devoted to his old buddy but is at a loss when he can no long "kid around" with the person with Alzheimer's disease. Many people are embarrassed to deal with or discuss the nitty-gritty of the patient's personal care.

You may find that you are still playing out the same major life roles in your relationship with a person who is no longer the same, but former communication habits may no longer be viable either. For example, some people are accustomed to using sarcasm as a way of relating dissatisfaction; Alzheimer's victims cannot understand sarcasm. Others are reluctant to discuss feelings yet it is often impossible to decipher the Alzheimer victim's feelings without thoughtful and creative questioning. Some individuals are totally undone by confrontation, criticism, or voiced anger; the person with Alzheimer's often cannot keep himself from acting in an angry and abusive fashion.

At this juncture, you must seriously consider whether old habits are interfering with good communication between you and your loved one. It may be very difficult to change, but the consequences of not changing ineffective communication patterns will increase the difficulties of being a caregiver.

Hidden Feelings Influence Communication

You may find it increasingly difficult to communicate effectively, not only with your loved one but also with others around you. There are good reasons for this. For one thing, the difficulties of the situation in general may be provoking strong negative feelings in you that you bring to communication encounters. That is to be expected. These feelings are normal. You may not even be fully aware that you are carrying them around with you.

Questionnaire II lists some of these common and expected feelings. Rating yourself honestly on this chart may help you identify feelings that are preventing positive communication.

First check the answer that best describes each of your feelings. Then add the numbers of the ratings you chose. If your total score on Questionnaire II is 75 or higher, you might benefit from talking to a trained counselor or consider getting some help from a support group, psychologist, or psychiatrist to work out these feelings. If your score is below 35, make sure you have added correctly or are being honest with yourself.

Questionnaire II
HIDDEN FEELINGS THAT INFLUENCE COMMUNICATION

	Never or Rarely 1	Some-times 2	Frequently but Decreasing 3	Frequently and Increasing 4	All of the Time 5
Guilty					
Angry					
Confused					
Helpless					
Ready to Give Up					
Out of Control					
Isolated					
Blaming Others					
Needy					
Financially Strained					
Resigned					
Desperate					
Lonely					
Self-Blaming					
Frustrated					
Neglected					
Numb					
Depressed					
Tired					
Uninformed					
SUBTOTALS					

TOTAL (all 5 columns) ☐

Questionnaire III

TOUGH COMMUNICATION SITUATIONS

Rate each situation from 1 – 5 according to the following scale:

> RATING SCALE
> 1 – Relatively easy, not a problem for me
> 2 – Occasionally difficult, but I do it
> 3 – Moderately difficult, I'd rather avoid
> 4 – Very difficult, but not impossible
> 5 – Impossible

Rating	Situation
_____	Asking for help from family members
_____	Asking for help from professionals
_____	Entering into conflict with other family members
_____	Entering into conflict with the person who has Alzheimer's disease
_____	Exerting influence over others, attempting to get them to agree
_____	Talking about certain subjects such as personal hygiene, details of illness, abusive language, death, autopsy
_____	Sharing information with professionals and people who work for me, such as homemakers, previous acquaintances, other caregivers
_____	Giving support, encouragement, praise out loud to Alzheimer's victim
_____	Seeking support, encouragement, praise from others for myself and for the person with Alzheimer's
_____	Accepting support, encouragement, praise from others
_____	Explaining my decisions and actions to others
_____	Describing my own needs, fears, problems
_____	Talking to my support group
_____	Explaining Alzheimer's disease to children, grandchildren, others
_____	Inviting people to my home

Ineffective Communication Tactics

Another reason for sudden difficulties is a common one. As your relative's communication abilities deteriorate, you may find yourself developing some ineffective tactics for dealing with him. This happens to people even with the best of intentions. Below is a list of responses to your relative that are not unreasonable or unusual. Such responses, however, may actually contribute to a further breakdown in communication between the two of you.

His Problem	*Your Response*
He doesn't seem to understand conversation.	You say less.
He doesn't respond to questions the first time they are asked.	You yell louder, thinking you'll get through somehow.
He repeats and repeats.	You simply ignore him.
He asks you a question for the tenth time.	You tell him to be quiet; you know he won't remember the answer anyway.
He uses a wrong word.	You correct him right away, hoping he won't make the same mistake again.
He needs to have a task explained a dozen times.	You do the job yourself and save both of you the bother.
He embarrasses you at your neighbor's house.	You stay home.
He has come to depend on you like a child.	You talk to him like a child.
He can't seem to remember the names for common objects, such as salt or sugar, even though you know he still knows them	You withhold objects until he says their names, hoping it will force him to maintain his vocabulary.
He "rattles on and on" all day long.	You play the radio or TV all day to drown him out.
He can't stay on the topic of conversation.	You let him go on and on, "tuning him out."
He is slow to understand and respond.	You "help" him by pushing him along and speaking for him
He has difficulty getting an idea across.	You distract him by changing the topic or engaging him in a different activity.
He gets impatient and frustrated because he doesn't understand.	You let him know that you are just as impatient and frustrated and can hardly stand it any longer.

Tough Communication Situations That Caregivers Face

In your role as caregiver you will face very tough communication situations. Questionnaire III lists several encounters in which you are likely to find yourself. Some may be new experiences for you. This chart will help you pinpoint situations that may be especially difficult for you personally.

Some of these tactics are ineffective for obvious reasons. If your loved one is not hearing impaired, yelling will only rattle him and add to his confusion. Treating him like a child or infantilizing him will only make him all the more dependent and warp your relationship further.

The reasons that other responses are ineffective or even harmful may not be so obvious. Removing communicative responsibility from the person with Alzheimer's in any way – by filling in words, by eliminating social contacts, by relieving him of tasks he is still able to do – forces him into further isolation and reduces effective communication prematurely.

Quashing attempts your loved one makes at communication by ignoring him, shutting him up, or correcting him constantly will only take away his desire for communication. Adding noise or unusual demands (such as "Tell me the name of what you want before I give it to you") to the communication environment usually proves distracting and disturbing.

If you find you are using several of these tactics, do not despair. Chapter Three discusses how to cope with the diminishing communication skills of the person for whom you care. It presents several techniques to help you with getting through.

Keeping in Touch With Yourself and the World

Several years a commercial about Al-Anon, the support group for relatives of alcoholics, was shown on television. It ended with these words: "You can see what his alcoholism is doing to him. Can you see what it's doing to you?" Replace the word "alcoholism" with "Alzheimer's" and ask yourself the same question.

Alzheimer's has been described as a disease of separation that results in losing a person in bits and pieces. Caring for someone who is dying this slow death over a period of years is more stressful than anyone who has not experienced it can imagine. Your loved one's needs are increasing daily. What you may forget or even not realize is that, as his needs for support increase, so do yours. It is important to know that his needs are NOT more important than yours. In fact, it is probably the other way around because the caregiver is the one who "keeps the show going." The caregiver must maintain her strength.

Maintaining communication with yourself and the outside world can help sustain you through difficult times. Remember that human beings *need* to communicate. Communication can give us strength. It brings us "comfort and inspiration" and helps us achieve our goals. The authors' experiences have shown that whatever her "communication style," the caregiver's own needs for interpersonal communication become greater, not less, as the disease of her loved one progresses. To ignore these needs can have disastrous results for the whole family. Beyond your communication with the Alzheimer's patient, it is crucial that you find ways to keep in touch with yourself and with the outside world. Communicating with and understanding yourself and your needs, knowing how you feel physically and emotionally, is essential if you are to maintain your equilibrium. You need to make time for yourself. Time for relaxation. Time alone. This is true whether you are home all day or continuing in a job outside the home. You must make time to communicate with *you*. If you focus all your attention on the patient and cease to be the person you once were, in the end you will both be lost.

Communicating with the outside world is equally essential. During this difficult time, communication with people outside your home can be especially beneficial to you.

There are people who can give you advice and suggestions for managing your situation, help you in planning the future, give you recreation and enjoyment and provide emotional and psychological support. There are even people who can help in arranging care so that you can get out of the house to meet all these communication needs.

Who are these "outsiders?" They are the other people in your family, old friends, neighbors, Alzheimer support groups like the Alzheimer's Disease and Related Disorders Association (ADRDA), nearby religious or civic groups, and local professionals, such as doctors, social workers, home health care aides, and so forth.

What can communication with these "outsiders" gain for you? For one thing, they can help you obtain precious time away from the person with Alzheimer's disease. No matter how strong his dependency, no matter how reluctant he is to let you out of his sight, you need time away. Your physician, social worker, or local chapter of ADRDA may be able to help you find an adult day care program for your loved one or a home care aide that you can afford. Keeping your sanity is worth the financial investment. If those options are not available, ask a friend or family member to spend a few hours with the patient on a regular basis. A caring replacement brings a fresh perspective and may actually improve the situation for everyone concerned. You should not feel reluctant to ask for help. It may be one of the most unselfish things you can do.

If you find yourself in a situation in which none of these standard relief caregivers is available to you, you are still not without options. One caregiver contacted the Catholic Newman Club of a nearby college and arranged to have "two strapping young male volunteers" provide several hours of care per week. She felt confident in their commitment and ability to handle any situation, and eventually they became "like nephews" to her, enriching her life as well.

Instructing surrogate caregivers can be difficult, however. After all, nobody knows your loved one as well as you do. Nobody else understands how the disease is affecting his behavior. No one else could possibly know how to use the successful management techniques that you have developed through trial and error over time. It is therefore crucial that you become able to communicate successfully and clearly with replacement caregivers so they will be effective and you will have peace of mind. (Some suggestions for succeeding with the difficult communication task of instructing surrogate caregivers can be found in Chapter Five.)

Once you have freed some time for yourself, you can reexamine your needs, get back in touch with yourself and your feelings, and take advantage of other benefits that "outsiders" can offer.

There are many people you can approach for advice and suggestions on the business of caregiving. For example, a good lawyer can be a supportive ally in preparing legally for the inevitable future. A financial consultant may also be helpful. If your physicians are experienced in treating Alzheimer's patients, consult with them often about your concerns. (Suggestions on how to communicate effectively with lawyers and doctors can be found in Chapter Five.)

You also owe it to yourself to seek out old friends and have a good time once in a while. Go to a movie or out to eat without the Alzheimer's patient. Accept an invitation to a party, a play, or a concert. If no one invites you, invite someone else. Take in a quiet museum, a game of golf, or just a pleasant drive. You might even consider joining or rejoining an organization you enjoyed in the past, such as the garden club, the Elks, the swim club, or the library league. It will do wonders for you spirits and put you back in touch with the world outside your home. Remember that you will not be taking care of your loved one forever. The grim reality is that in a matter of a few years you will be on your own again. It is important to maintain your contacts. Remember too that the better you feel, the better you will be able to minister to your loved one while he is with you.

The most significant thing that "outsiders" can give you is emotional and psychological support. Support groups like ADRDA put you in touch with other people who are living through the same experience and understand how difficult your situation is. Learning how other people cope and sharing your own discoveries and feelings can be enormously helpful. Nationally affiliated support groups can give you a wealth of good information and suggestions that can take some of the stress out of your caregiver job.

If you are feeling especially depressed or anxious, or if the diagnosis of Alzheimer's disease has stirred up old tensions that prevent your family from functioning effectively, you should consider meeting with a professional counselor, psychiatrist, or psychologist. Your physician, social worker, or ADRDA can recommend one. Counseling is not necessarily expensive. Many mental health centers operate on a sliding fee scale, and some health insurance plans partially or fully cover short-term counseling.

Counseling for the entire family may help relieve emotional strain, isolation, and interpersonal tensions. Although it may not be easy to convince some family members that counseling would be helpful, it is worth a try.

You can keep yourself in touch with the world outside even on those days when you are not able to get out. Telephoning or letter writing can be helpful in meeting your communication needs. Write a letter to a friend you have not seen in ages. Call and make plans for a future outing. Telephone your daughter who lives in another city. Whatever you do, maintain your contacts.

Chapter Three
GETTING THROUGH TO EACH OTHER

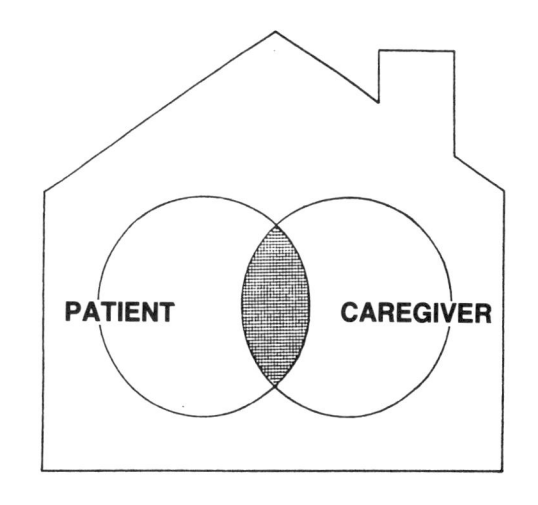

Improving the Bonds of Communication

The first two steps toward improving the bonds of communication between you and your loved one are the treatment of the "other conditions" described in Chapter One and the emotional preparation of you, the caregiver, for the job at hand as discussed in Chapter Two. Chapter Three deals with the third component of the communication model, the actual communication that occurs between you and your loved one. This chapter describes how to identify specific communication barriers and sets the stage for getting through. Strategies for successful communication encounters are presented to assist you in four basic areas:

- developing ways to get and maintain your loved one's attention;
- learning to use the kinds of language that get the best results;
- using activities as a means of encouraging communication; and
- knowing what kinds of communication are best for reducing undesirable behaviors.

Many suggestions that follow may seem like small steps to take in attempting such a difficult task. Taken together, however, they have a powerful effect on the overall communication process.

Remember that some of these ideas will work well, and some may not work at all in your situation. Others may work one time but not be very successful at another. From this smorgasbord of options you will be able to choose the strategies most effective for your particular loved one at her particular stage of the disease. You are the expert on your loved one. Only you really know her and what works best for her. Furthermore, it is you who must put these steps into action. You are encouraged to consider each suggestion and its appropriateness for your loved one, giving each idea at least one good try.

Getting and Maintaining Attention

One of the biggest problems in getting your message across to the Alzheimer's patient is getting her to pay attention to what you are saying. Although little can be done to restore the actual powers of concentration, you can take many steps to make the most of the attentional abilities that remain.

Keep in mind how hard the Alzheimer's patient has to work to make sense of what is going on around her. Distractibility is a primary problem. When there are competing visual, auditory, or other signals, she has great difficulty determining which ones are the most important. Therefore, the first step in getting her attention is to remove as many distractions as possible. The person will do best when she is dealing with only one signal at a time.

In a global sense, this means your loved one's environment and routine should be simplified whenever possible. A confusing home life fosters confusion, and confusion leads to stress. All persons have difficulty maintaining attention under stress, but it is especially difficult for persons with Alzheimer's to focus their attention on any one thing when their environment is cluttered and noisy. If the daily routine is irregular with many unexpected interruptions, the patient is likely to be in a chronic state of distraction.

For these reasons, your communication is more likely to be successful if the message you are trying to get across does not have to compete with other messages. If you are trying to say something important, be sure the TV or radio is off and other people are not talking at the same time. Do not try to convey information while your loved one is concentrating on doing something else like taking a bath or riding the bus or tying her shoe. You simply will not get through.

When you want her to pay attention to what you are saying, be sure she is tuned in before you begin. Position is also important; make sure your loved one is facing you when you speak. This also adds visual cues to your message that help her focus on what you are saying. You may also want to change your body position in relation to hers before you begin to talk. If she is standing, keep her in front of you as you speak. If she is seated, bend over or sit next to her so she can see you easily at her eye level. Avoid approaching her by touch or voice from behind; she does not process unseen signals as we do. They startle and confuse her, making her less able to receive your message.

A number of other devices can be used to enlist her attention before you begin to speak. Call her name; touch her on the arm or face. Take her hand to help her focus on what you are saying. Change the pitch of your voice. If you talk in a lower tone of voice, for example, it will alert her to tune in to what you are saying. Talk more slowly. Talk a little louder. No matter what, *never begin to speak without first getting her attention.*

Make your message as graphic and clear as possible. For instance, if you are asking her to brush her teeth, demonstrate by "brushing" your finger across your teeth while you make your request. Using gestures will often make what you say more easily understandable. This simple tactic will save you both time and energy and prevent needless frustration.

Making Language Work— Getting More Out of Less

The Alzheimer's patient has many problems processing language messages. These difficulties in understanding spoken language generally stems from deficits in four basic areas:

- memory function
- comprehension
- linguistic skills
- social communication (pragmatics)

By understanding why your loved one has problems with language in a particular situation, you can more easily employ a number of strategies to compensate for these difficulties. Specific techniques are listed in the chart on pages 28-29. There is some overlap because one strategy may help compensate for several deficits. The efficacy of these strategies has been verified in research by the authors and other scholars.

Beyond the specific suggestions presented in Chart II, there are some general principles to keep in mind that will make language work better for both you and your relative.

Avoid Interrupting

First, *try not to interrupt* the person with Alzheimer's disease when he is attempting to get an idea across to you. If you interrupt him while he is talking, he is likely to lose his train of thought. That will make him feel all the more out of control even if he is not sure why he feels that way. Your interruption also communicates to him a certain disregard or lack of respect for what he still has to say.

Be a Creative Listener

In order for your companion to be most successful in communicating his ideas to you, you will need to do more than simply listen without interrupting. First, you will want to *be a "creative listener."* Instead of reacting to his actual words, you must learn to read the "subtext" of his message and interpret what he actually means. Try to get at the thought or feeling underlying what he is attempting to say. Look for cues in his facial expression, tone of voice, and behavior. Sometimes when you interpret and rephrase aloud what the patient has said, or state for him what you think is the underlying feeling that might have prompted his words, you will be surprised that he is able to tell you whether you are on target.

Your willingness to listen and help may reassure him and in turn eliminate some of your own frustration. For example, a demented person who repeats over and over, "I'm tired. I'm tired." may really be trying to say, "I'm frustrated, I don't know what to do with myself. I may as well go to bed. There doesn't seem to be anything else I can do anymore." A sympathetic "I'm sorry you're so frustrated," is a more appropriate response than "So go to bed!" A statement such as "Where is my mother?" may represent a feeling of insecurity or fear. Responding with "Don't worry, I'm here to take care of you," may reassure him and allay some of his fears.

The following passage from *The 36-Hour Day* illustrates the helpfulness of making an effort to interpret your loved one's statements.

A family member contributed the following interpretations of the things her husband often said. Of course, we cannot know for sure what a brain-impaired person feels or means, but this wife has found loving ways to interpret and accept the painful things her husband says.

He says: "I want to go home."
He means: "I want to go back to the condition of life, the quality of life, when everything seemed to have a purpose and I was useful, when I could see the products of my hands, and when I was without the fear of small things."

He says: "I don't want to die."
He means: "I am sick although I feel no pain. Nobody realizes just how sick I am. I feel this way all the time, so I must be going to die. I am afraid of dying."

He says: "I have no money."
He means: "I used to carry a wallet with some money in it. It is not in my back pants pocket now. I am angry because I cannot find it. There is something at the store that I want to buy. I'll have to look some more."

He says: "Where is everyone?"
He means: "I see people around me, but I don't know who they are. These unfamiliar faces do not belong to my family. Where is my mother? Why has she left me?"

In coping with remarks such as these, avoid contradicting the person or arguing with him; those responses may lead to a catastrophic reaction. Try not to say "I didn't steal your things;" "You *are* home;" "I gave you some money." Try not to reason with the person. Saying "Your mother died thirty years ago will only confuse and upset him more."
(Mace and Rabins, 1982, page 106)

In general, arguing with an Alzheimer's patient in nonproductive at best. If it does not bring on a catastrophic reaction or violence, it will surely lead to confusion for him and frustration for you. If you must voice your anger, be sure you send out "I" messages to state your feelings rather than "you" messages that will upset and discourage your companion. Say "*I* am so angry because I have to clean up this mess!" rather than "*You* made this mess on purpose. *You* just want to make me miserable. *You* have ruined my life!"

<u>Watch What You Say</u>

As you see the deterioration of your loved one take place, it is easy to believe that the per-

Chart II

MAKING LANGUAGE WORK: GETTING MORE OUT OF LESS

	MEMORY	**LINGUISTIC SKILLS**
EARLY "FORGETFUL" AND MIDDLE STAGES	• repeat messages frequently • use short sentences • ask one question at a time • break down instructions into separate components; give one directive at a time; e.g., "Put your arm in the sleeve." "Button up." "Tuck in your shirt tail." • provide written cues as reminders because written messages are retained longer than spoken ones; select *one specific place* where they are kept • give directions as close to the time they must be followed as possible (within an hour rather than the morning or the day before) • give directions in person rather than over the phone; supplement your directions with brief written instructions • remind him where he is and what time it is	• avoid asking open-ended questions, such as "What do you want to drink?" • offer two choices whenever possible: "Do you want coffee or soda?" • remember that word recognition lasts longer than word recall; say aloud what you think he is trying to say to see if he can signal whether you are correct; play "twenty questions" • use "fill in the blanks" to help him "find" the words: "Pass the bread and ____." • encourage circumlocution or "talking around" what he is trying to say • avoid correcting "wrong" words • allow him to write or spell words he cannot say • avoid interrupting or rushing him; allow him time for processing and understanding • look for clues to his message in his facial expression, tone of voice, behavior
LATE STAGES	• remind him tactfully what he was talking about during conversation • make such things as familiar music, pictures, scents available to him	• use a reassuring tone of voice with lots of touch and body language; he may still understand a wave, an outstretched hand • avoid saying things in his presence you do not want him to know; it is impossible to know how much he understands

Chart I

LANGUAGE BREAKDOWN IN PERSONS WITH ALZHEIMER'S DISEASE

EARLY "FORGETFUL" AND MIDDLE STAGES

COMPREHENSION

LANGUAGE BASED:

- repeat message frequently
- use simple words
- use short sentences; avoid using complex sentence structures
- ask one question at a time
- break down instructions into separate components; allow time to finish one task before moving on to the next
- supplement spoken with written language
- paraphrase a sentence when you repeat it; use synonyms
- enhance your message by using pictures, objects, gestures, body language

ATTENTION BASED:

- avoid competing messages, such as television, radio, other conversations; anticipate difficulties in large groups or with strangers
- speak slowly
- speak face-to-face, making eye contact
- use appropriate tone of voice for your message; avoid sending unintentional emotional signals by your manner of speaking
- use a calm, pleasant tone of voice so that he wants to tune in; avoid addressing him as a child

SOCIAL COMMUNICATION

IN CONVERSATION:

- keep him on the subject by asking relevant questions
- keep the conversation going by offering your own associations to his remarks: "That reminds me of the time..."
- summarize what he has said in a conversational way
- avoid difficult social situations, such as those with strangers or groups
- encourage simple social interactions in which he can be successful and those for which his language skills are sufficient, such as close friends, relatives
- orient him to upcoming situations; tell him what is about to happen: "Your sister Mary is coming to visit." "The doctor is going to examine you now."
- be as reassuring, respectful, and affectionate as possible so he *wants* to communicate with you

---

LATE STAGES

- assume there is some substance in what he is saying if he attempts to communicate
- listen to his jargon; it might give clues
- ask him to repeat
- guess at his meaning

- continue to offer interaction, conversation
- maintain social rituals, such as greetings, saying goodbye, and so forth
- prevent withdrawal as long as possible by continuing to interact with him; don't stop talking

son you once knew is no longer "there." It is also easy to fall into the casual practice of speaking in front of the individual as if he does not exist. You may find yourself telling graphic stories of how he has gone downhill, how difficult he is to care for, how he used to be so brilliant and capable of so many things. Remarks such as these are often related in detail by caregivers to others in the presence of the person with dementia.

Avoid discussing the person in his presence as if he were not there. Although you need to vent your feelings, choose your moments and your audience carefully. Sound off when your loved one is not with you. Although his comprehension of verbal messages regresses, the person maintains, mysteriously at times, an acute awareness of the mood, tone, and attitudes of those around him. If he hears you discuss him, he will inevitably receive the message that he is a failure and at fault for all your troubles even though he did not understand the meanings of the words you said.

The Alzheimer's victim is frequently depicted in a frightening series of pictures as an attractive woman fading further and further from view. However, until the most severe and final stages, persons suffering from dementia experience what has been called "windows of lucidity." These are true, if fleeting, moments of understanding. You cannot predict when they will happen. How sad for him to have such a flash of insight just when he hears you angrily deliver a very explicit message about him to someone else.

Keep Talking

A final point. To make these suggestions work, you must *keep talking* to the person with Alzheimer's disease. Techniques such as these will not be helpful unless they are used consistently. No matter what your "personal communication style" was before your loved was stricken with Alzheimer's disease, you must continue talking to your relative as much as possible to keep the communication process alive.

Creating Success

Positive communication is found not only in words but in so much that is beyond words. In the following pages a number of other channels through which you can send messages of love, caring, and interest will be described. If you make it a point to look for and create times for him to feel successful, he will be getting a comforting and supporting message and you will be "getting through."

Using Verbal Praise

Especially in the early stages but also in lucid moments throughout the illness, the person may be acutely aware of failing and failure. At the same time, childlike, he can be tremendously pleased at the tiniest achievement. The ability to recite the names of grandchildren, tie a bow, or finish a meal will bring a beam of triumph to his face.

Develop a sixth sense for these moments. Openly acknowledge them with a responding smile, touch, or praise. Your obvious approval is very important in staving off impending fear or panic and in reassuring the individual that he still has value and worth.

People normally do not pay much attention to such small things because routine behaviors seldom attract much attention. To praise a person for finishing his juice or making it to the bathroom without an accident may seem patronizing or ridiculous. But one has only to recall the struggle required for the person with dementia to stay on task, even briefly, to recognize the significance of such an accomplishment. Communicate your appreciation of such efforts frequently and honestly. (You are, after all, pleased he made it to the bathroom. It has saved you a lot of work!)

Using the Sense of Touch

Touching is the most important tool for communication you have, right to the very last moment of your relationship with this person. Touch speaks eloquently either to enhance your words or to replace words altogether. A pat, a small hug, a brush of the hair, a stroke, a guiding tug, holding hands, or resting a hand on the arm of your friend or relative as you minister to, talk with, or simply sit next to her communicates your message. Each gesture is a gentle and persistent way of saying "I care," "I'm here," "Pay attention," "I can help you," "This is the way," "You're not alone."

In infancy, one of the earliest needs is for bonding by physical contact. It is also the final need. People never lose their hunger for the nourishment that comes from the touch of others. Experiment generously with the number of "touching messages" you can give in the course of a single day. Notice if her behavior changes in response. Watch your own positive feelings change and grow as you communicate in this way.

Using People: Children, Grandchildren, Friends, and Relatives

The coordination of children's needs and perceptions with those of the rest of the family can be a monumental task in itself. Add to the equation a relative with Alzheimer's disease, and you can be completely overwhelmed. Communicating effectively at these times requires a delicate choice of words and a sensitive attention to nonverbal messages.

Shaping Attitudes Through Words and Actions

Children, for the most part, are very resilient. What seems to you a harmful exposure to unpleasant or unnatural circumstances can become a growth and maturing experience for the child. Your attitude and method of explaining why Grandmother or Aunt Alice behaves oddly will almost totally shape how the child reacts and behaves around her.

Be frank and honest without providing so much detail or graphic description about the condition that the child is frightened. Describe the illness in a way that maintains the dignity of the loved one. Read, for example, the very warm and wise explanation of Alzheimer's disease offered by one adult to a small child in *The 36-Hour Day:*

One father put a pile of dried beans on the table. He took little pieces of the pile away as he gave his young son the following explanation of his grandfather's illness: "Grandpop has a sickness that makes him act like he does. It isn't catching. None of us is going to get like Grandpop. It's like having a broken leg, only little pieces of Grandpop's brain are broken. He won't get any better. This little piece of Grandpop's brain is broken, so he can't remember what you just told him; this little piece is broken, so he forgets how to use his silverware at the table; this little piece is broken, so he gets mad real easy. But this part, which is for loving, Grandpop still has left."

(Mace and Rabins, 1982, pages 151-152)

Talk to children about "illness," "needs our help and love," and the necessity of a calm and reassuring tone of voice when talking to your relative. Choose words like "unusual" or "unexpected" rather than "weird" or "crazy." Discourage the child's use of derogatory and value-laden terms as well. Appeal to the child's sense of creativity by asking for ways he might better be friends with or of help to Grandma.

If the children live in the same house as the Alzheimer's patient, avoid burdening them with endless "babysitting" responsibilities that could be tiring and frustrating to both individuals. Be aware that children too have a threshold for burnout and look for some outside counseling or support for them, if necessary. The people in your support group may have good ideas about helping children cope.

Children will also learn largely from watching the ways *you* communicate and interact with the family member who has dementia. Your role modeling is more important than any words of explanation you can offer. Nowhere do actions speak louder than words than in a situation like this.

Arranging Visits

Grandchildren may live far away or there may be former students or neighborhood children of whom she was especially fond. Visits from children are special, but these youngsters may not be familiar with the course of the disease and the personality changes that are taking place. Still, this is not a good reason to discourage them from stopping by. Let them know that you would like to see them and invite them for a certain time and day. Tell them you are not able to have guests "pop in" unexpectedly. Wisely prepare them for the changes they are going to see. Grandchildren will probably stay longer, but a brief visit (5-10 minutes) from other young friends may be all that is necessary.

Rather than excluding children because you fear embarrassing moments, include children in your routine, whenever possible. Children can become your allies in creating chances to refresh and revitalize your loved one's interactions with others. Above all, you are setting up additional opportunities for healthy communication.

What about visits from friends and other relatives? The reality is, others are sometimes frightened and uneducated about how to interact with this person they no longer know. Recall that when the disease first manifested itself, your reactions were different than they are now. Through experience you have learned to expect the unexpected, a lesson friends and relatives have not yet learned. You cannot force others to visit, of course, but to defend yourself and your loved one from isolation, you may to choose to "educate" others about the disease and its effects.

If you feel unsure about doing so, here is a suggestion: Start with an especially close friend, your minister or rabbi, or an understanding neighbor. Take some time to discuss your situation and describe some of the ways your relative responds best when others are talking to her. Next invite that person to come over for a brief visit and ask him or her to try consciously to use the same approaches you have found successful. Explain that it could take several visits to feel truly comfortable.

Today, thanks to the amazing grassroots efforts of the Alzheimer's support groups, most people have at least heard of the disease. But Alzheimer's disease still bears an aura of mystery and fear, and much of the education of others lies in the hands of you who truly live what has been called "the 36-hour day." It is you who are educating the professionals; it is also you who must educate your friends and relatives.

Using Activities

Activities, especially familiar and favorite ones, are a rich resource for communication. Activities give you the opportunity to talk about what you are going to do, talk about what you are doing, and then talk about what you did. You may learn that activities that once gave pleasure or ones that she previously did very well may still be possible in a modified or shortened form. For the person who enjoyed baking, for example, a simple task such as mixing batter with your close supervision could be quite easy for you to set up, yet very rewarding. An individual who formerly engaged in woodworking activities could, for a time, still sand or lacquer with a little help. You will discover that using simplified activities based on the person's previous hobbies, employment, or life style can create quality time for you to spend together.

Whether gardening or caring for house plants was an earlier hobby, this activity may have great therapeutic value now. Gardening provides exercise and a variety of stimuli through texture, aroma, and sight. Because different seasons produce differing growth, gardening is also a good tool for marking the months of the year.

Communication during any activity will deteriorate quickly if you do not first take a few precautions. Set a certain time, perhaps 10-15 minutes, that keeps in mind the other person's attention span and your own limited time and patience. Choose tasks that have only a few steps and guide the person through each step, one at a time. Avoid activities that require any new learning or skills.

Music, Rhythm, and Exercise

Most people develop an early and deeply felt enjoyment of music and rhythm just as they do for touch. Music is pleasurable, soothing, and therapeutic. Like touch, music can send messages in a way far superior to words. Old tunes may evoke fond memories; light but lively rhythms can increase blood flow and oxygen to the brain and provide a good stimulus for a mild exercise program. Humming softly as you help bathe or dress your relative can sometimes quiet her anxiety.

Rummage through old record or sheet music collections; ask a music store dealer for suggestions of quiet, calming music; or secure a hymnal from church. Try playing soft music, especially in the late afternoon and evening or on gloomy, cloudy days to reduce the "sundowner" effect. Music can help you channel increased anxiety levels that cause more agitation. Steve Halpern's (1979) cassette tapes are excellent for these times.

Record albums of old familiar tunes are also good for reminiscence. Your relative may sometimes be able to sing the words to familiar songs long after most spontaneous speech is gone. You might try tape recording certain favorite selections from these albums onto a cassette tape. For many, the button on a tape recorder is easier to manage than following all the steps necessary to get a record or compact disc player going.

If you do have taped music that she enjoys, experiment by having her listen to the tape recorder through earphones which can be purchased inexpensively from most electronics stores. Listening with earphones focuses the sound more clearly and reduces other distractions. This will also provide you with a few bonus moments of quiet. Avoid suddenly descending on her with a menacing-looking pair of earphones, however. First plug them into the tape player and put them on yourself to demonstrate how they are worn. Adjust the volume control to a comfortable listening level. They lay them on the table and invite her to try for herself or place them gently on her head if she will allow it.

There are some lovely videotapes available (Windham Hill, 1984) that show breathtaking scenery against a background of soothing music. If you have a video cassette recorder (VCR), you can rent these tapes for a small fee in almost any video rental store. If this pleasant sight and sound method is successful in calming your relative or friend, you might consider purchasing the tape as a Christmas or birthday gift. The one entitled *Water's Path* is a favorite.

A light program of exercise for persons with Alzheimer's is considered essential by most professionals. You play your part in encouraging this activity by joining in and leading the movements. The music and exercise together provide a nice communication bond for the two of you, and no words are needed. Records or cassettes that have a light easy rhythm are best. Exercise might also be more fun if familiar music is used. Your resource for more information about music and exercise is a recreational therapist* or an occupational therapist.*

Pets

Pets are another potential source of pleasure, and they are fun to talk to. People will often speak to pets even though they may avoid talking to other people. Pets are unassuming and friendly and the good feelings that come from stroking their fur or watching them move about is calming and reassuring. Pet therapy is now recognized as a valuable method for combating depression and withdrawal, especially among the elderly and lonely. Pet therapy plays a major part in many counseling or specialized residential settings. Many dentists have found that an aquarium of colorful fish in the waiting room calms the anxious patient.

If you do not already have a pet, be cautious about acquiring one at this time, however, Dogs and cats, especially, may best be purchased when they are young, but their friskiness, plus the discipline and attention that a new pet demands, may disrupt the routine of a household that is already in delicate balance. However, some pretty fish or a small bird could be a nice and less demanding addition. You may have a friend whose pet you can "borrow" or visit on occasion if you have none of your own.

If you do already have a pet, you can use it to create situations in which the person with Alzheimer's is doing the caring instead of being the one cared for. Brushing, feeding, changing water, or walking with the pet under supervision can provide a valuable sense of involvement and usefulness.

Language Exercises
In the Early Stages

1. Crossword Puzzles: If your relative enjoyed doing them before, working crossword puzzles can be a pleasant way of keeping her active and stimulated. Choose very simple ones. Do half the puzzle one day and half the next. Keep it fun. Do not let it become a drudgery or a frustration. Use "choice" questions " Do you think they mean a mule or a cow?") much of the time when you know the answer and she does not.

2. Categories: Ask her to name...an animal, color, shape; something round, hot, soft; something you might find in a closet, in a hardware store, in your purse. Ask him... when we wear swimsuits, gloves, or tuxedos; when we wash our hands, change a tire; or put gasoline in the car.

3. Humor: Get a book of limericks, riddles, or jokes from the library. Together figure out the play on words and discuss why they are funny.

4. Word Games: Stimulate her recognition of words with the old standard games, such as"Hangman." Do the "Jumbles" in the daily newspaper or create your own "jumbles" or "word searches" using names of famous people and places or other interesting words.

5. Coupons: Sort shopping coupons into categories. Begin with an index card for each category (beverages, cosmetics, cereals, and so on). Use the pictures to locate items in the grocery store.

6. Time Games: Purchase a large cardboard clock, sometimes found in a children's toy shop or a teacher's supply store. Review "What time do you...?" Have her fix the hands of the clock to the correct time then write it down.

7. Problem Solving: Develop a list of practical considerations of everyday living, such as "What would happen if we...Left the stove on? Ran out of gas? Went outside without a coat? Became lost downtown?" Review these practical situations and their solutions often.

In the Middle Stages

1. Labels: Make labels using index cards and large easy-to-read letters written with a felt tip marker. Tape them on appliances and containers that store important items.

2. Current Events: Cut out several prominent newspaper headlines and their accompanying photos. Help your relative match each headline to its photograph. Discuss why they go together.

3. Phone Numbers: Have her dial important phone numbers, matching the number written on a card to the dial. Or across a plain piece of paper, write out your own telephone number in large fat print. Write a matching set of numbers and cut each one out. Ask her to match the cutout numbers to the telephone number on the paper. Encourage her to do this in sequence to help her retain the actual telephone number.

4. Family Photos: Have her match written names to photographs of family members. Practice naming photos of distant relatives. Discuss the events that surrounded the occasion of the picture taking.

5. Copying: Have her copy her name and other words in block letters, saying the words aloud together.

6. Comics: Read aloud the daily or Sunday comic sections of the newspaper together. Talk about the humor in each strip.

7. Sorting: Have your relative put away items from the grocery store while naming

them and talking about them.

In the Late Stages

1. Play favorite songs and sing with her at bedside.
2. Reminisce while bathing or dressing her.
3. Use parallel talk, telling her what she is doing while she is doing it.

The Life Review Diary

The following activity, the Life Review Diary, was first developed by Lynn J. Holland, Ph.D. (1984), in her work with nursing home patients who have dementia. Dover (NJ) General Hospital has also used a modified version with Alzheimer's patients still living at home and their families with gratifying results. The life review process is based on the premise that reality for the person with dementia is the world of past, not current, experiences. Reality is *within* the person rather than what is going on around or outside the person. Short-term memory is fading or gone. The "now" is often confusing, meaningless, or scarcely recalled. Past experiences become the "stuff" of which this person's world is made and are retained, however fuzzily, almost until the end.

The Life Review Process highlights the individual's distant memories and uses them constructively. By completing the sections of the Life Review Diary together and only a little at a time, you and your loved one can recall the past and validate its importance.

If possible, as often as every day if you can, choose a section in sequence to the one most recently finished and read it over to her. Take time to explain questions not understood. Stop to ask questions specific to the information. Allow her time to recall other memories. This activity is not meant to be a drill session in memory. It should be treated as a relaxing moment when the past is given its due. During this time, her seemingly endless and perhaps wandering recollections are totally permissible and patiently shared. Though it may not always be practical, try to complete one section of the diary in a sitting. If she has the tolerance, review some of the first page each time. To "set the stage," reconstruct present biographical data at the beginning of your session. One additional use of the Life Review Diary is to tape record each section and encourage her to listen to the memories during quiet or just-sitting times. The hearing and rehearing of her life's most significant moments can serve to renew and reinforce that ever-elusive sense of self and reality.

Dealing with Difficult Behaviors

What behaviors are unpleasant and desirable? Why, in fact, is a section on difficult-to-manage behaviors included in a book about communication?

Some examples of undesirable behaviors that often irritate, frighten, embarrass, or exhaust the caregiver and friends are abusive, argumentative, insulting, or complaining language; catastrophic reactions related to seemingly unimportant events or changes in routine; "stubbornness" or refusal to cooperate; repetitive questions or actions; pacing or wandering; uncontrolled shouting; incontinence; and hallucinations. Coping effectively with such behaviors calls for your best communicative efforts.

When these behaviors occur, you need to be alert to both the *verbal* and *nonverbal* meanings that the person with dementia is trying to convey. At these times your skills as an interpreter are especially crucial. The success you have in dealing with these situations will depend, in turn, on the skill and control with which you deliver your verbal and nonverbal messages.

Prevention

Possibilities for both prevention and limitation of some unpleasant behaviors will be discussed in this section. Nonverbal and verbal strategies discussed in detail elsewhere in this book are summarized for you as follows:

Prevention: Nonverbal Strategies

- Keep your daily routine simple and stable.

Life Review Diary

THE AUTOBIOGRAPHY
OF

_____

Today I am going to write about myself, my life and times.

My name is _____. The town I live in is _____. My address is _____. The phone number is _____.

At home, my room contains some of my own things, such as _____
_____
_____

My most frequent visitors are _____
_____
_____

Of all the possessions I have, the one that gives me the most pleasure is _____
_____

My favorite song is _____

I'm sentimental about _____

Things that make my life complicated or frustrating are _____
_____

What I like most about myself is _____
_____

I forgot to mention _____

My best advice to young people is _____
_____
_____

MY CHILDHOOD

I was born in _____

on _____

I am the son/daughter of _____ and _____

They came from _____

There were _____ of us in our family then. My sisters were named _____

_____

and my brothers were named _____

_____

We lived in _____ until I was _____ years old.

My favorite memories of childhood are _____

_____

_____

I went to grade school in _____

To get to school, I had to _____

_____. My favorite teacher was _____

_____, and my favorite subjects were _____

_____

I had to memorize _____

_____

The games I learned to play were _____

_____

My best friends were _____

_____

I was very good at _____

_____

My first sweetheart was _____

My pet was named _____

37

MY TEEN YEARS

I grew and changed from thirteen to nineteen. I learned to _____

_____

I lived in _____ with _____

I developed into a quite a nice person. My hair was a _____

color, and I wore it (how) _____

In my day, everybody wore _____

I always liked to wear _____

My favorite color was _____. The popular song of the day was _____

_____. My hobbies were _____

_____

My friends and I liked to _____

One time I remember we got into trouble because we _____

_____

My education _____

I earned money by _____

_____

People gave me compliments because of my _____

_____

I was proud of my _____

_____

I could always depend upon _____

_____

My favorite teenage memories are _____

_____

_____

_____

MY LIFE AS A YOUNG ADULT

In my twenties and thirties, there were some big changes in the world around me and in my own life; some of these were _____

_____

_____

_____

Some new opportunities for me were

Family changes: _____

_____

Living in a new place: _____

_____

New skills and interests: _____

_____

New neighbors and friends: _____

_____

Most of my time was spent _____

_____

I could always depend on _____

_____

These are some of the memories of myself as a young adult: _____

_____

_____

_____

_____

_____

_____

MY MIDDLE YEARS

After I turned forty, it seemed that my life changed in some ways and remained the same in others. My life was still _____

The major changes in my life were _____

My biggest challenge was _____

I learned how to _____

I was especially proud of _____

People noticed that I could _____

I could always depend upon _____

My family life _____

If I could give just one bit of advice to a person of forty, it would be _____

Some of my favorite memories from my middle years are _____

PRIME TIME

Since I turned sixty, the major changes in my life were _____
_____
_____
_____

Right now, these are the things making my life complicated or frustrating: _____
_____
_____

but I know that next year all that could change.

These past few years I've made quite a few discoveries about myself and my life: _____
_____
_____

I have developed some new strengths: _____
_____

Some new skills: _____
_____

Some new friends: _____
_____

And some new ideas, too: _____
_____
_____

What I like most about myself these days is _____
_____
_____

I still depend upon _____
_____
_____
_____

If I could wish one wish for this world, it would be _____

_____

This coming year, I plan to _____

_____

_____

_____

Date completed _____

Assisted by _____

- Reduce household hustle and bustle. Noise and distraction may tend to agitate your loved one and lead to catastrophic reactions "over nothing."
- Keep both yourself and the patient in good health.
- Keep yourself in reasonably good mental health. Your calm and reassuring attitude will have much to do with successful preventive care.
- Wait for his responses. Allow sufficient time for him to understand and follow instructions whenever possible rather than jumping in and saying or doing for him.
- Rely on his poor memory. If he refuses to go somewhere or do something that must be done, leave your request for the moment then return to it later as if it were a new idea. Change your tone of voice; rephrase the goal or destination.
- Encourage him in small tasks of very short "do-able" steps and limited duration to help him feel wanted and useful.
- Become well-informed about and cautious in the acceptance and use of chemical restraints, such as tranquilizing drugs.
- Consider physical restraints only as a last resort. Speak first with your physician and understand fully the types of restraints available, their use, and the effects they can have on the person.

Prevention: Verbal Strategies
- Frequently praise and reward acceptable behaviors.
- Remember to address him directly, face to face, and always use a comforting touch as an added message.
- Your words to him should be simple and truthful. Avoid the kind of teasing that can confuse him and bring on stubbornness or refusal to cooperate.
- Ask him to do one thing at a time, not several. Practice breaking one task into several little steps at which he can be successful.
- Speak to him as an adult, not as if he were a child.
- Avoid pressing him to remember something he cannot, even though you feel he should. If you can see he is having trouble finding the words, use some of the verbal strategies already described to help him think of what he is trying to say.

Limiting or Stopping Unpleasant Behaviors

Realistically, you will not be able to avoid all unpleasant situations, in spite of your best efforts. Your first line of defense is recognizing why the person in your care exhibits these undesirable behaviors. It is not because you have failed. It is due to the brain deterioration. As the disease progresses, he has less and less control over his brain function.

If the behavior in question is not characteristic of the person's day-to-day behavior, consider that the problem may be due to an undetected medical condition. Stomach aches, constipation, low-grade fevers, impacted earwax, or a toothache can cause sudden onset or escalation of pacing, night wandering, incontinence, or yelling. Consult your physician about these and any other unusual behaviors.

Your more immediate, on-the-scene responses to the undesirable behaviors are of great importance. Your goal, when these upsetting occasions arise, is to prevent escalation of these behaviors and stop them altogether as quickly as possible.

Limiting or Stopping: Nonverbal Strategies
- Obtain a Medic Alert bracelet immediately. The bracelet should say "Memory Disorder." Other people need to know your loved one's condition, should you not be present. (The address of Medic Alert is listed in the Appendix.)
- Whenever possible, district him by placing something in his hands to hold, carry, or otherwise manipulate. Ask him to "help" you with something.

- Guide him to a less public place if you can.
- You may try to ignore certain behaviors, such as repeated questions or abusive or insulting language. If you do, keep in mind that this type of behavioral management is not yet well-documented as a successful method for decreasing unpleasant incidents in persons with dementia. Make sure you are absolutely consistent with your ignoring. Know enough about yourself to recognize your own suppressed anger at these times. Try again to divert your companion to a more positive activity or conversation.

Limiting or Stopping: Verbal Strategies
- Keep your messages short, firm, and uncomplicated. During a catastrophic reaction you definitely wish to be understood.
- Rely on your tone of voice even more than your words to convey a calm assurance and firm control. If he hallucinates, denying his statements probably will not work and may even lead to unsettling arguments. Change the subject, distract him, or offer to "check it out" together. At the same time, offer calm reassurance that you are there to make sure everything is going to be all right.
- Above all, avoid verbal arguments. They are easy to fall into, especially in moments when the person has forgotten what he has just said and now says the opposite, denying his earlier statements.

Involving Others: A Good Idea

Early in the course of the disease, you may it is "too soon," "too embarrassing," or "unnecessary" to speak openly to friends, neighbors, and relatives about the unpleasant behaviors your loved one is beginning to exhibit. Nevertheless, you will find it is never to soon to include these people in your plan for prevention or limitation of undesirable behaviors.

Involving others is truly an act of safety made in the interest of the Alzheimer's patient. By preparing friends and relatives, you are giving them the means to deal with uncomfortable or emergency situations now and in the future. Furthermore, you are relieved of the heavy burden and strain of trying to hide sad, frightening, or embarrassing knowledge.

Explain to friends and relatives that if they meet with such behaviors as wandering or blunt accusations, their gentle but firm reassurance, distractions, touch, and calm guidance are *their* best tools for handling unpleasant situations, just as they are yours. Above all, reassure them that these behaviors are not to be taken personally. Encourage them to read parts (or all) of this book so they too can become confident in their approach to communicating with your friend or family member during difficult times.

Coping with the Blind Alzheimer's Patient: A Special Challenge in Communication

If you care for an Alzheimer's or dementia patient who is blind, maintaining meaningful communication can be especially difficult. Although the important visual channel for getting through to the other person is closed, the following modifications and extensions of ideas found elsewhere in this book will help you communicate more effectively. Suggestions of professionals to contact for help with special problems have also been included.

Focusing Attention

Gaining and retaining the attention of the blind confused individual can be difficult. Because he may be able to distinguish vague shadows, always be particularly careful to address the blind person from the front. This tactic reduces startle and fear reactions and more effectively focuses attention on you and your message.

Touch is also an especially powerful method for getting the blind person's attention. Furthermore, touch also doubles as an important communication bond between the two of you. If your blind relative is highly resistant to being touched, however, you may have to begin a regimen of desensitization. Desensitization is a method used to accustom a person gradually, one step at a time, to being near or touching something they formerly could not tolerate. If you need help, an occupational therapist* can assist you in developing such a program.

Use of Speech, Language, and Voice

All the recommendations on pages 28-29 that do not require the use of pictures, labels, or written messages are particularly critical ones for you to follow when you communicate with your blind relative. For instance, you will be more effective in getting through to him if you use brief, simple sentences. You need to be especially cautious about identifying yourself when you approach him and naming or describing objects or actions that are part of your activities together.

To improve communication, work at modulating your voice so the intent of your message is clear. This means using a lot of expression, keeping your pitch low, and speaking slightly louder than normal without shouting. With the blind person it is truly not so much what you say as how you say it.

A speech-language pathologist* who has had special training in using augmentative communication methods can show you how to supplement talking with other ways of communicating. The speech-language pathologist is a good resource in helping you discover other means of getting through to your relative.

Movement and Balance

The blind and confused individual will probably also have special movement and balance difficulties. He may also be highly resistant to and fearful of unfamiliar or unexpected physical contact. This can make giving helpful guidance to him a special problem, particularly when it is necessary to take him out of the house. A physical therapist* can advise you about using a wheelchair at these times and getting your relative accustomed to this unfamiliar means of conveyance.

Home Environment

There are a number of changes you can make in your home that will make communication between you and your relative easier. Consider placing rails on some of the walls, perhaps from his bedroom to the bathroom. Consult an occupational therapist* about these and other special safety measures, such as the use of iridescent tape and brightly colored carpet squares. These details and others can make it easier for you to persuade him to move about and keep active.

Using bright lighting enhances communication because it reduces depression. It also increases the individual's ability to see and understand gestures and other visual cues. Bright lighting is especially important when the Alzheimer's patient is blind because many blind people can distinguish light from dark. They can detect the presence of a shape or shadow when someone or something is in front of them. By keeping your house brightly lighted, you will help the individual be better able to sense your approach and focus on your presence.

Activities

Rhythm, music, exercise, children's voices, and pets may be some of your best resources for keeping both harmony and mental stimulation in your loved one's life even though he is blind. You should not scrimp on these resources. Use them often and in as many ways as possible.

Using and discussing familiar scents is also an excellent activity to use with the visually impaired individual. Textures are also a good source of stimulation. When the Alzheimer's patient is blind, you can supplement or replace visual activities by presenting a variety of textures, such as finger paint, playdough or clay, lotion, crackly cellophane, and so forth for him to explore.

Keeping the avenues of hearing and listening actively involved is also important. Tapes, music, radio, and television, if used judiciously (that is, not blaring constantly), will help keep the blind person in communication with the world and with you. If you need more ideas, a patient activities coordinator* (sometimes known as a recreational, music, or art therapist) can be creative in helping you learn how to stimulate and communicate more meaningfully with the blind confused person.

Further assistance may be obtained by contacting your state's Commission for the Blind. It should be listed in the white pages of your local telephone directory. The Commission may also be able to refer you to healthcare professionals in your area who are skilled in working with the blind and elderly disabled person.

Chapter Four

GETTING THROUGH TOGETHER: THE COMMUNICATION ENVIRONMENT

Home

The home environment needs to be safe, secure, and orderly for the person with Alzheimer's disease. The home is also the primary communication environment and the fourth component of the communication model for *Getting Through*. Although some home environments greatly encourage communication, others can actually discourage or prevent it. It is important to be sure that your home is not working against your efforts to maintain effective communication.

Lubinski (1981) described what she called a "communication impaired environment" as "a setting in which there are few opportunities available for successful, meaningful communication." The communication impaired environment is one in which the physical design of the setting inhibits comfortable, private conversations; where noise, television, and traffic also inhibit talking. A communication impaired environment has poor light, poor acoustics, and is unfamiliar, unstimulating, and unsupportive.

Your first concern, of course, must be to keep your home safe, secure, and orderly. This serves communication needs as well. When your loved one feels secure and safe in familiar surroundings, he is better able to concentrate on communicating effectively. There are many things you can do to help. You can enhance his sense of security with the use of written cues and labels around the house. Clearly written notes not only help to maintain your relative's sense of order but stimulate memory and language use as well. Simple reminders to "turn off the water" or "step up" can add to this security. Labels on such items as the kitchen appliances and canisters may help forestall loss of some specific words in his vocabulary.

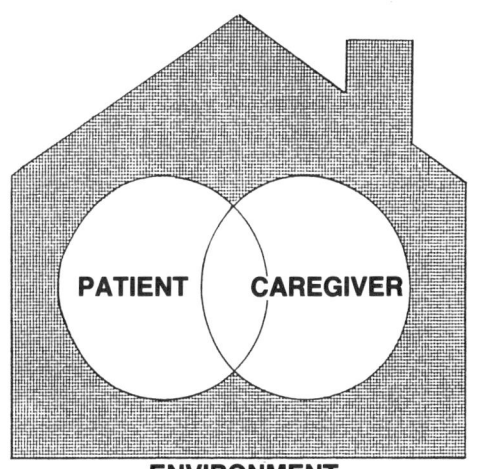

Even though you need to remove or lock up many household items to guarantee safety and security, it is important that the house remain stimulating. Interesting pictures, especially photographs of familiar people, should remain in view. Activities that stimulate language use and communication, such as playing cards, jigsaw puzzles, and pets, should be available.

Lighting in the house should be strong enough so that visual communication cues, such as facial expressions and written directions, are not missed. Bright light can also help prevent anxiety and depression on cloudy days. Clutter should be removed to avoid distraction. A telephone with an amplified speaker should be obtained if your companion has any difficulty hearing.

Above all, the home environment should have a comfortable place for talking and people to talk to. The "talking place" should be the same one it always was. If important family discussions always took place in the kitchen, conversation should continue there. If you enjoyed quiet talks on the front porch, you should still have them there even if you must put up gates to make it safe. Continue to invite those people who regularly came to talk. Keeping the home conversation going is a pleasant way of "getting through."

Adult Day Care

If you find that you and your loved one are becoming increasingly isolated and uncommunicative in the home, or if your loved one is now requiring more supervision at home than you are able to provide during the day, consider taking him to one of the many adult day-care centers that have been established in recent years. Adult day-care programs provide a wide range of social, medical, recreational, therapeutic, custodial, and supervisory services. A good day center will not only care for your relative in a secure environment; it will also keep him busy while giving you, the caregiver, respite and support services. Often, such programs can help you postpone the permanent placement of your loved one in a nursing home.

In choosing an adult day-care program, you should look for all the same environmental factors that keep your home from being "communication impaired." Is it quiet? Are the lighting and acoustics good? Is it safe? Is it stimulating? Is it clean and comfortable? Are there people with whom your loved one will want to communicate?

Communicating in the Nursing Home

You may find, as many families do, that you can no longer care for your Alzheimer's relative at home and must consider moving him to a nursing home. As your experience with placing a relative in the nursing home begins, you will find yourself face to face with a new set of challenges. Among these is the need for both you and your loved one to shift into different communication roles to match your changed communication environment.

This shift presents a tough set of demands. You will better adjust to these demands if you are familiar with some typical communicative situations that can occur in this setting. If you are aware of potential conditions or needs, you are better equipped to deal effectively with them.

To ease adjustment to this new environment you can look at these communication roles in terms of the situations the two of you must meet *together,* the kind of communicative environment *your relative* will meet in the new place, and the changing requirements for *you.*

Preparing to Go

If your loved one retains any comprehension of language or events, you will have the difficult task of somehow breaking the news of the move to her. So much is involved: Her poor memory erases your explanations immediately; the disease-induced suspiciousness and dependency make packing a major chore; and your own mixed emotions may seem to paralyze you. Some families have even resorted to telling the individual they were going to take her to visit someone in the home and then left her there. Despite problems in communicating, your relative deserves a better introduction to her new residence than that.

If you have the luxury of time and proximity...and if she will tolerate riding in a car and is not too difficult to transport, drive to the home several times to familiarize her with her new surroundings. Take a photograph and refer to it positively and frequently during the next days or weeks. If she can still read and understand single printed words, attach a label the picture with the words NEW HOME written in large print.

Actually visit the residence too if this seems reasonable. Even without the personal visit, however, familiarizing her with the photograph(s) may help focus her attention on the event. Can she help you pack in some way? How about allowing her to help select the personal items she is going to take? If she can take part in these tasks, she may feel more in control of the move she must make.

There is the risk, of course, that her comprehension of the upcoming move will cause more problems than a lack of understanding. Comprehension brings with it anxiety and a confusion of feelings. She may barrage you with questions and accusations that make you feel miserable. Not knowing how to respond when she asks: "Why are you putting me

Step of putting patience in the home.

there?" "When can I go home?" "Why do you want to get rid of me?" increases your own anxiety. You will need to reassure her continually and let her know you still care for her.

Pattern your answers to her questions so that *you* maintain responsibility for the move. Instead of telling her "You're too sick to stay home any more" or "You'll have a lot more friends there," keep your explanations in the form of "I" statements. Say: "*I* am not able to care for you any more." "*I* am not strong enough to lift you." "*I* don't seem to be able to do it all by myself." These kinds of "I" statements avoid blaming her and keep you in control of the move, whether or not you like it.

Often, persons are transferred directly from an acute care hospital to the nursing home when, for medical reasons, they can no longer live alone with their families. If she is not well, she may not put up the same resistance, but she will still need the same verbal and nonverbal explanations and reassurances. These pave the way to better adjustment later, no matter how useless they may appear at the time.

Arriving at the Home

In the first moments, hours, and days she will encounter an exhausting number of new communicative situations. Some that you can meet together are making introductions to her new roommate; lunching for the first time in the community dining room; meeting the direct-care nursing and aide staff; greeting other residents; and meeting a new physician.

Decide how to keep in frequent contact as she begins the gradual process of adjustment to the nursing home and its routine. Phone calls, little notes, a tape-recorded message, and visits are all ways of communicating to her (and to yourself) that she has not been deserted. The choice, of course, depends on how close you live as well as on the routine of the home. Ask the nurses for other ideas on how best to maintain contact.

Keeping in Touch with Each Other

One of the things that can become very tiresome is keeping up the burden of communication that, by now, may definitely have become a one-way street. It is difficult to take the total responsibility for maintaining a positive but sometimes one-sided relationship. As a result, one's visits may become shorter and less frequent. They may seem awkward and even pointless.

However, there are several positive ways to prolong a sense of communication between the two of you. One is by giving some prior thought to your visits so they do have more quality and worth, even if your idea of what is meant by "worth" must change with the changing condition of your loved one. Visits can be planned around the various kinds of *communication* that still have meaning for both you and her. For example, you can:

- Bring new pictures for her photograph album and talk about the events surrounding the picture taking.

- Arrange to have a telephone hooked into her room and make a couple of calls to grandchildren. Since numbers and dialing may be confusing, and phones are not readily accessible in most rooms, this could be a real treat.

- Tape record a family mealtime, religious service, or social occasion (five minutes may be long enough) and bring the tape to her for listening, either together or for later when you have returned home.

- Write short notes to friends and relatives with her. Address Christmas cards or other types of greeting cards. Such gestures may stimulate others to return the kindness.

- Residents who wander often find companions who do the same. Walk together with them for a while. You will learn, as they may have, that the need for companionship and communication does not always include the need for words.

- Occasionally bring an item from home that she is unable to keep at the nursing home; talk to her about it and remind her of the

pleasure she once derived from it.
- You need not bring gifts on every visit, but an occasional small token is a wonderful way to say you care, are still interested, and think of her. Alternate your gift ideas, if possible, between items you can enjoy together during the visit and ones that can occupy time or memory after you have left. Some lotion to rub on dry hands and legs is a good example of the former. A small tin of aromatic tobacco or a ceramic night light with a little drop of perfume on the bulb might be nice for the latter.
- Check the nursing home's schedule for conversational topics that center on her new life. These should also be a reminder that you may sometimes join an activity with her. Song fests, church services, or exercise time, if permitted, can be pleasant times for you to be together without talking.
- Express your love verbally, simply, and often. Watch for even fleeting expressions in her eyes or gestures that let you know she is aware you are with her and likes it. You will not want to miss that moment.

Your Relative

The magnitude of changes that the communicative environment in a nursing home brings should not be overlooked or underestimated as you observe how she is getting along. Her ability to communicate effectively without a lot of support is already greatly reduced due to the course of the disease itself. Poor health, impaired hearing or vision, limited mobility, and side effects of drugs are all factors that compound the problem.

These factors are *internal* to the person and her state of being. Given that the individual has already become a poor communicator, what can be expected from the environment in which she is going to reside? What are the *external* factors, those that relate more specifically to the nursing home setting itself? Can a residential home, even under the best of circumstances, support and encourage quality communication between staff and patient or resident and resident? The reality, of course, is that it does not; it cannot.

In 1981 three researchers in speech-language pathology assessed the communication atmosphere in one nursing home in New York City (Lubinski, Morrison, and Rigrodsky). They spoke to over forty residents in one wing of the home to obtain the patients' own perception of the quality of communication. They asked the residents to whom they spoke, how often, where, and about what topics. Although the researchers were careful to point out their findings were made based on the study of only a single setting, their general conclusions are thought-provoking and apply to many residential settings.

They found that the institutionalized setting can represent the epitome of the "communication impaired environment." The residents in this study complained of a perceived lack of activities to generate interesting conversation; an attitude of the staff that promoted a "serene" environment – the "good" patient is the quiet patient who gives the nurse little trouble and takes only a small amount of her time; of long hallways that discourage easy movement and architecture tiresome to look at and navigate; and of the lack of quiet rooms where residents could have private conversations.

The high rate of staff turnover in many nursing homes also reduces opportunities for bonding and intimacy between nursing staff and patients. This rate can be as high as 40–50% a year in a "good" nursing home. Many aide positions are filled by persons with limited proficiency in English, individuals who have only recently immigrated from other countries or who are from socioeconomic backgrounds that do not place a high value on "unnecessary" social communication.

Without making any value judgments about such conditions, one has to accept them as they are. Be aware that institutions by their very nature create many barriers to communication. As changes in the quantity and style of your relative's communication occur, you need to compare these changes to the atmosphere in which she now lives. It will then be up to you to decide whether advocating for different conditions would be practical.

You

Being a relative or friend of an institutionalized person is a new role for most people. Don't be surprised if you need help to cope with making the decision to place your relative in a nursing home and with the new type of "getting through" required. There are several positive ways to build and maintain good communication with both the staff and the administration to deal more effectively with some of the gloomy realities described above.

Naturally you want your visits to make a difference to the person you have placed in the home. But when that is no longer a possibility (and even before), you must revise your expectations and accept that other avenues of communicating can have great value instead.

Support Group

If the nursing home has an advocacy or advisory committee or support group (better yet, a support group designed for relatives of patients with dementia), join it. In time, what you gain from this association can prove as valuable as your interactions with the nurses who care for your relative. Several studies have shown that when residents' families participate in groups that share experiences, receive information, or advocate for change, their acceptance of a relative's nursing home placement is significantly better. As a result, the quality of family-resident interaction is also improved.

"Re-entry"

Once your relative has been placed in the nursing home, balance "re-entry" into your former activities with care and foresight. On one hand, getting out and enjoying yourself refreshes your outlook and is definitely recommended. However, a headlong rush to fill the newly empty minutes can quickly become an unconscious defense against the pain of visiting your relative or friend. Allow yourself time so that being "too busy" does not become a routine reason for not going to visit.

Connecting with the Staff

Make a conscious effort to seek out the nurses and aides who have primary responsibility for your relative. They are your most vital link to the nursing home and your loved one. Learn when it is best to call or speak to them so that they are not in a rush at the time of your contacts. Try to reach them at that same time each week or at regular intervals. They will appreciate your consideration of their busy schedule, and if they are expecting your call, they will be more likely to have the information you want.

Connecting with the Administration

During your initial fact-finding visits to the nursing home, you should become comfortably acquainted with one or two of the administrative staff, This will serve you well in the coming months and years when you may want to iron out other matters and solve any problems that may arise. Disagreements and complaints between your relative and the staff are likely to happen. Do not be too inclined to brush these off as the paranoia that usually goes with dementia. Refrain from blaming the staff or institution before you have the facts, however. If problems do arise, make appointments to see administrators only after you feel you have both sides of any complaint concerning your relative. Always seek the opportunity to settle such issues by communicating with the direct-care staff first.

Avoid starting such discussions when you happen to catch an administrator in the hall. You will want the administrator to give you their best attention; this can be accomplished most easily by seeing the administrative staff in their offices at an appointed time. Begin your discussion in the light of constructive problem-solving and seek solutions in a spirit of compromise. Your tactful efforts to communicate should have a positive payoff for both you and your Alzheimer's relative.

Chapter Five

COMMUNICATING AS A CONSUMER/ADVOCATE

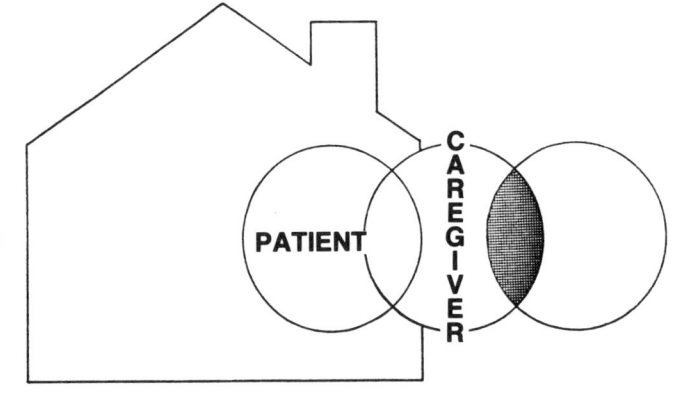

Knowing What to Get; Getting What You Need

A consumer uses a product or service. An advocate acts in someone's behalf to make conditions better. In healthcare a "consumer/advocate" is one who looks for the best quality of healthcare services available and then tries to make them even better.

Take the active role of healthcare consumer/advocate for the good of your loved one. If you are going to be effective, you must be perceived as a healthcare consumer who wants to learn and be informed. You must be able to communicate with the service providers with whom you come in contact and ask the right questions. It is much easier for the professionals with whom you meet to respond to issues you bring up than for them to anticipate your unvoiced needs.

To help you communicate with these professionals, several sets of questions are presented for you to draw upon during your interviews with physicians, attorneys, home health aides, and nursing home administrators. The suggested questions were prepared with the assistance of key members from each of the professions. Every question on each list was carefully considered and included for a specific purpose. They address those matters you need to learn more about in order to make better informed decisions.

You may wish to do some background reading on unfamiliar topics before your meeting. Feel free to ask each professional to explain their answers if you are unsure of the meaning, either at the time of your discussion or afterward. If the person sitting across the desk from you does not have or cannot get most of the answers you are seeking, you probably need to look for someone else who can better serve your needs. You must feel free to get a "second opinion" if you are told, "Oh, that doesn't apply in your case." It really may not, but check it out anyway if you feel uncomfortable.

You may be wondering if you should actually sit in the office of a perfect stranger and begin reeling off questions with pencil and paper in hand. Yes and no. These questions are certainly not meant to be used as a hostile tool that makes you look suspicious or places you in an offensive position. What they do is provide you with an excellent starting point, a "talking paper." It is perfectly all right to carry them with you to help you remember what you want to know. It shows the professional that you are concerned about your loved one and have "done your homework" for the interview.

Bringing someone else with you to take notes may also be a good idea. That would leave you free to talk and absorb the information. Studying the questions, writing the answers, or bringing a friend or relative for support is the kind of thoughtful planning that can make you a more successful healthcare consumer/advocate as well as a respected communicator.

Remember, you have the right and responsibility to choose the best qualified professionals to help you provide quality care. The following guidelines will enable you to make informed decisions confidently about the professionals and services you select.

GETTING THROUGH: COMMUNICATING WITH YOUR PHYSICIAN

What you want to obtain from your family physician (general practitioner or internist):

- Orders for series of in-depth laboratory tests. (Approximately 15% of diagnosed dementias are now known to be potentially reversible. Since Alzheimer's disease is not presently treatable, the physician will want to be sure before saying, "There's nothing we can do." The tests listed in number 2 below comprise a minimum test battery to rule out other conditions which may mimic the symptoms of Alzheimer's.)
- A referral to a neurologist or a neuropsychologist for further confirmation of the diagnosis.
- Treatment for any treatable medical condition or referral to the appropriate specialist.

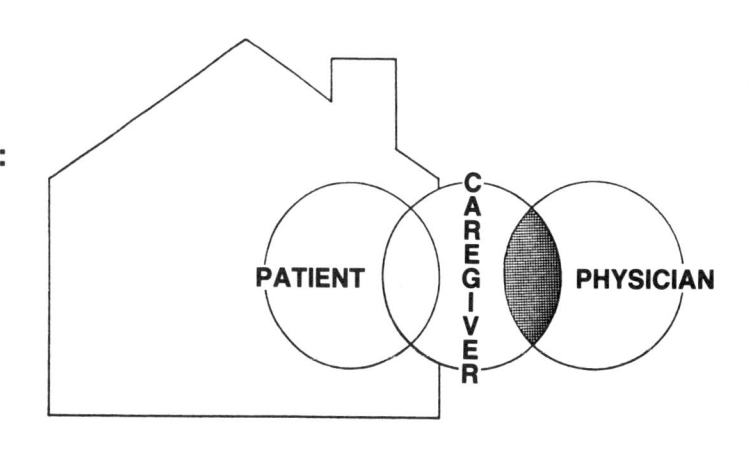

COMMUNICATING WITH YOUR FAMILY PHYSICIAN

1. Doctor, we understand that senility or severe memory loss is *not* an expected part of normal aging. Could you order a complete series of laboratory tests to rule out other causes for my relative's changed behavior?

2. (After the tests:) What results did you find in the
   complete blood count (sedimentation rate)? _____
   standard metabolic screening? _____
   thyroid function tests? _____
   vitamin B-12 and folate levels? _____
   urinalysis? _____
   serologic test for sexually transmitted diseases? _____
   CT scan? _____
   electroencephalogram (EEG)? _____

3. Do you suspect Alzheimer's or some related disease? _____

4. (If so:) Can you refer us to services or persons in our community who can help us? _____

5. We want to make sure we have covered every possibility. Can you also recommend a neurologist (or neuropsychologist) to us? _____

6. If your physician wonders why you "want to put her through all of this," respond that:
   You would like to know for genetic reasons,
   You would find it easier to know what you are coping with, or
   You need to know in order to make other family decisions.

7. May we have a copy of our relative's medical history to take to the other doctor(s)? _____

8. What medicine has been prescribed? (Write down the name of the drug.) _____
   How soon can we expect to see some positive changes? _____
   What are the possible side effects that could occur? _____
   _____
   Has the drug been approved by the Food and Drug Administration (FDA)*? _____

9. (If she will enter a nursing home:) What is her level-of-care rating? _____

10. We will ask the neurologist (or other specialist) to send you his report. When would you like to see our relative again for another checkup? _____

11. (If this is a follow-up visit:) What changes have you noticed? _____
    _____

What you want to obtain from the neurologist (or neuropsychologist):

- Results of neuropsychological testing, preferably conducted twice (two visits separated by a period of at least six months) to detect cognitive decline and mental deterioration.
- If the family doctor has not already ordered them, the neurologist will see that a CT-scan, an electroencephalogram (EEG), and possibly a spinal fluid analysis are done. (The latter test is by no means universal. Physicians are cautious about using an "invasive" technique – in this case, drawing fluid from the spine – if a satisfactory diagnosis can be made without it.)
- After ruling out all other possible causes, a relatively definitive diagnosis of Alzheimer's disease or some related disorder may be expected.
- In some cases a medication may be prescribed to reduce incontinence, night pacing, agitation, or depression. (The neurologist should serve as a resource to the family for monitoring the effects of any medication.)
- A description of community resources and healthcare professionals who can offer help, support, and information or the telephone number of your state's ADRDA office. (The national ADRDA office address and telephone number may be found inside the appendix of this book.)
- At least one follow-up visit.
- A report sent to the referring physician (your family physician) and to any other specialists you designate.

COMMUNICATING WITH THE NEUROLOGIST

1. What are the results of the tests? _____

2. What do you think she has? _____

3. (If Alzheimer's disease or a related disorder is suspected:) At what stage (how far along) do you think she is? _____

---

*Experimental drugs should only be used in a controlled study conducted in an approved research center. One should not have to pay for experimental drugs.

4. What can we expect now? What is the course of this disease? _____

5. Are there any other medical specialists whom we can consult regarding care for other conditions? _____

6. How can we maintain her present level as long as possible? _____

7. What medicine has been prescribed? (Write down the name of the drug.) _____

   Is this an experimental drug or has it been approved by the FDA? _____
   What are the possible side effects of this drug? _____
   (When a drug is prescribed, it does not mean it is going to work; adjustments in type and dosage are to be expected, especially in Alzheimer's patients whose drug tolerance is often unpredictable.)
   When may I call you about the need for drug adjustments if her behavior changes for the worse?
   _____

8. How soon should we make another appointment? _____

9. Whom can I call to learn in more detail about caring for an Alzheimer's patient? _____

10. Can you suggest anything for me to read? _____

11. What other services or resources (such as counseling, legal help, support groups, help at home, respite care, day care) are available for us? _____

12. (If this is your second visit:) What changes have you noted since our last visit? _____

13. (If the patient will be entering a nursing home:) What is her level-of-care rating? _____

Autopsy

At some time, usually when your relative is placed in a nursing home, the very delicate issue of autopsy should be explored. Alzheimer's family members may feel pressed to permit an autopsy for the purpose of furthering scientific research. They may also have fears, reservations, or religious objections about the autopsy procedure. Too often the subject of autopsy is taboo, however, and the decision whether or not to permit autopsy is not made until death is near. No matter what they decide, people may later be consumed by guilt or regret about decisions made in haste at a time of great emotional stress. For this reason, family members should learn their rights and make known their wishes ahead of time, not at the critical moment of death.

As uncomfortable as it may seem, you may want to ask your primary physician, neurologist, or attending physician at the nursing home the following questions:

1. How great is the present need for medical information obtained through autopsy of Alzheimer's victims? _____

2. If we decide to allow this procedure, how can we be assured that our relative's remains will be treated with respect? _____

3. Can I designate or have some guarantee that all the organs will be buried or cremated with my relative? _____

4. When is it customary to sign a consent for autopsy? _____

5. What if I change my mind at the last minute? _____

GETTING THROUGH: COMMUNICATING WITH YOUR ATTORNEY

Finding the Right Lawyer

Whether or not you have had much previous experience with the legal profession, you are sure to find those first sessions in the lawyer's office fraught with anxiety. You will be discussing issues that change people's lives – and the consequences of their deaths – and the responsibility is awesome. How best to get through, say what you mean, and find out what you need to know?

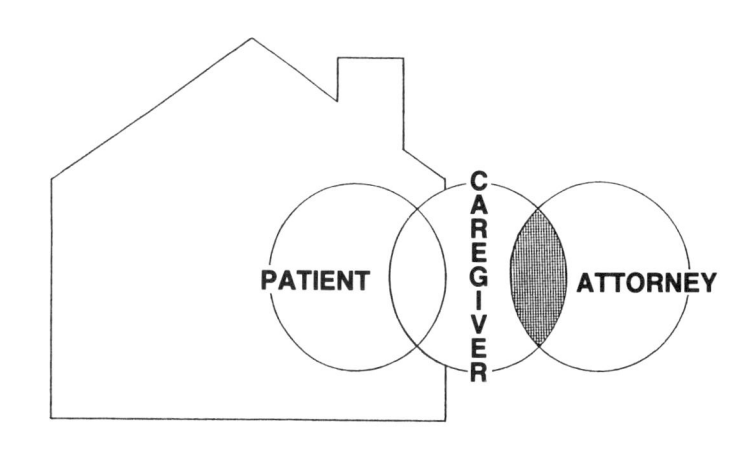

First, make sure you retain a lawyer who is a specialist in estates, retirement, trusts, government benefits, and the aging. Ask members of your support group or call your county bar association. They keep lists of lawyers who are specialists and can recommend two or three attorneys in your area.

Second, read over these questions and take them with you to the interview. Even though you may not understand everything on the list, a lawyer who is going to act in your best interests should. If you receive vague answers and too many promises to "look into that," consider looking further yourself. These matters are too important (and often, too expensive) to leave to just anyone.

Third, of the four professionals for whom guidelines are given in this book, the person with whom you probably have the greatest need for effective and long-lasting communication is your lawyer. It is crucial that the attorney you choose be skilled in making you feel comfortable, that trust be established, and that he be able to explain clearly all the intricacies involved.

Initial Information

(Over the telephone, probably to the receptionist:)

1. I'm looking for a lawyer who specializes in financial planning for persons who are elderly, mentally incapacitated, or institutionalized. Can you tell me if Ms. or Mr. _____ has had experience with families of persons with Alzheimer's disease? _____

2. What are your fees? _____
   (Initial visit? _____   Hourly rate? _____   By specific service? _____.)

3. How should I arrange for payment? _____
   (At the time of the visit? ____   By monthly bill? ____   Over several months? ____   At completion of service? ____)

4. If my relative/friend cannot leave the house or nursing home and I need to have documents signed in the presence of an attorney, would you be willing to come to my house (the home)? _____
   What is your fee for a home visit? _____

5. What documents or information should I have with me or be gathering for our meeting?
   Nursing home contract _____   Lists of assets and liabilities _____
   Patient's current will _____   Income tax return, previous year _____
   Documentation from physician or nursing home of necessity of medical (not just custodial or "convenient") home care? _____
   Power of attorney (if you already have one) _____
   Marriage license, divorce papers, other contracts _____

6. Can you furnish me with a list of what I need to make a thorough report of all assets and liabilities?
   _____
   _____

Guardianship and Conservatorship

1. What is the difference between a conservatorship and a guardianship? _____

   My relative is already totally unable to think or do for himself. Are either appropriate in our case?
   _____

   (At this point, the lawyer will probably ask to see your power of attorney, if you have one. A lawyer who is skilled in *geriatric law* will want to know if it is "durable.")
   If I must obtain a conservatorship or guardianship, how long does it usually take?
   _____

2. Will the court appoint a lawyer to represent my relative if my relative is opposed to this procedure?
   _____
   What is that attorney's function? _____
   Who pays that lawyer's fees? _____
   Must I, or my physician, appear in court? _____
   What kinds of questions must I answer? _____
   What will the fees be?   Lawyer _____   Court costs _____

3. If I'm appointed guardian, do I have the right to place my relative in a nursing home if he is mentally incapable? _____

4. If I am a legal dependent of the person in need of a guardian or conservator, can we word the petition that asks the court to appoint me as guardian or conservator so that I have the power to use a portion of my relative's assets (or income) for my own care as well as for the care and support of any other legal dependents? _____

5. Do I need to be declared a guardian or conservator in order to make decisions to terminate or withhold life-sustaining treatment when my relative reaches terminal stages? _____
   Or does this state allow the removal of life-sustaining treatment only if the patient expresses this desire explicitly while still competent ("Living Will")?

Durable Power Of Attorney

1. I have heard a *standard* power of attorney is not effective when my relative can no longer think or do for himself, and that a *durable* power of attorney means that the power of attorney is effective even after my relative becomes incompetent. How can I obtain a durable power of attorney? Could you show me in the document where those words are so I will know? _____

2. Specifically, what rights or legal obligations such as mortgage and transfer of property, taxes, insurance policies, and debts does this document cover? _____
What liability does this expose me to? _____

3. Does this paper include power over bank accounts, stocks and bonds, or safety deposit box contents? Or must I obtain a separate power of attorney for each of these from the individual institutions? _____

4. Does it give me the right to represent the patient before a government agency, for example, the Internal Revenue Service (IRS)? _____

5. Is it possible in this state to create a durable power of attorney that becomes effective only after total incapacity occurs? _____

6. If we decide to get a durable power of attorney, who makes the decision that he has become incompetent? _____ How long does this take? _____

7. Suppose my relative gets better, and we no longer want the durable power of attorney. Is it revocable? _____

Wills, Trusts, Taxes

1. Can you explain to me the legal rights and obligations of spouses (or any relative who has primary responsibility) in cases like ours? _____

2. Given our present and future financial situation, do you think it would be wise to set up a trust? _____ What are your fees for this service? _____

3. If we set up a trust, do we still need to make or revise a will? _____
Do I still need to obtain the durable power of attorney? _____

4. What is a "right of survivorship"? _____
Should we consider it? _____

5. Please list for me, step by step, what I must do to make sure my relative is cared for legally, financially, and medically, in case of *my own* untimely death. _____

6. Can I receive any state or federal tax relief if I hire someone to come into my home and care for my relative while I am working? _____

7. Given our present situation, do you think we need to be concerned with planning to minimize federal and state taxes? _____
   What steps must I take? _____
   _____

8. Should we consider declaring my relative a legal dependent of her child or of any other relative? (as in cases where direct payment of fees to the nursing home by a child or any other relative becomes tax-deductible) _____
   What steps must I take? _____
   What does this cost? _____ About how long does it take? _____

Medicaid, Nursing Homes, and Nursing Home Contracts

1. We are preparing to put our relative in a nursing home. Please go over the contract with me and explain any clauses that could have unexpected results later on. _____
   _____
   _____

2. The nursing home has told me that their contract is not negotiable. How does this affect my rights? _____

3. I am worried about what is going to happen when all our assets are gone. Are there any government programs in this state that might help me pay for the cost of medical care for my relative while he is in the nursing home? _____
   _____

4. Do my relative and I have to spend all of our joint (family) assets before my relative in the nursing home is entitled to Medicaid or any other government programs? _____

5. If my own income is over a certain level, am I still entitled to receive government or state assistance? _____

6. If my relative is eligible for government assistance, am I entitled to an amount of my relative's income for my own support (pension, social security, disability insurance) even though he is in a nursing home, or does it all have to be applied to the cost of care? _____
   _____
   What is an "order of support"? Do I need one to receive a portion of my relative's income? _____
   Is this expensive? _____
   How long does it take? _____
   What steps are involved? _____

7. To what extent is the spouse financially responsible for the support of the institutionalized spouse in this state? _____

8. What can you tell me about transfer of assets to others such as children, relatives, or friends before or after 24 months from the month of application for Medicaid? _____

Which assets are allowable? Which are not? _____

To whom may assets be transferred? _____

GETTING THROUGH: COMUNICATING WITH YOUR HOME HEALTH AIDE

A Visiting Homemaker Service is an agency that employs specially trained persons to go into the home and assist with personal, health, and light housekeeping chores. Qualified professionals such as registered nurses and medical social workers coordinate services and work with you to develop a plan of care. This team approach is called *respite care*. For a while, someone else takes over, and you are free to go out.

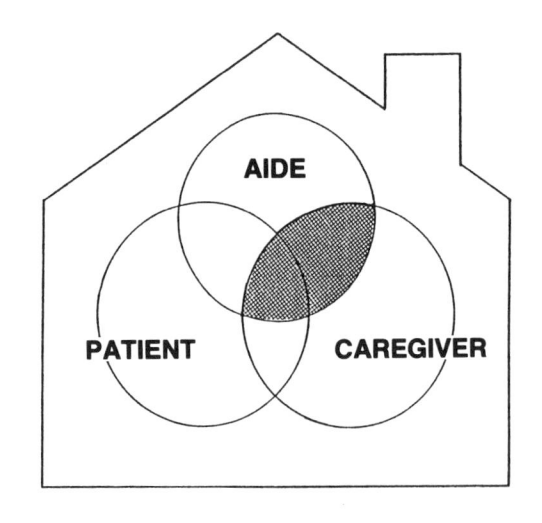

The communication role that you adopt with a home health aide is quite unique. When communicating with the lawyer, physician, or nursing home administrator, you must ask questions in order to make sound decisions, but the professional still "supervises" the situation. When first talking to a home health aide, you ask questions so that *you* can be the supervisor. And beyond that, you hope that you have found encouragement and companionship for your relative.

Many people have never had anyone else come into their home to work. Others have never supervised anyone in a job-related status before. Caregivers may also experience feelings of guilt about hiring someone else to do the work because "they'll think I'm lazy... don't love my father anymore... have a messy house... am made of money." They may even be embarrassed about Dad's behavior.

Another underlying fear is that "Dad will like the way she does things better than my way; she'll take my place." These feelings sometimes work to delay the caregiver from calling a home health service until things are at a crisis state. Arrangements may then be made between you and the agency that are unnecessarily hasty.

The lasting power of your business and personal relationship with a home health aide must focus on three areas:
- the *information* you obtain from your phone calls to an agency;
- the all-important *introductory meeting* (or interview) with the aide that you hold before you make a final decision to hire. It can take place informally between you and the potential home health worker or on the first official visit to your home, when he or she is accompanied by the supervisor; and
- your ability to tell another person clearly what caregiving steps are required, to *assist,* then *observe,* and *let go,* allowing the home health aide to do the job for which you have hired her.

Your First Phone Call

1. My relative has Alzheimer's disease. Does your agency employ specially trained persons to help out in such cases? _____

2. Is your agency a profit or not-for-profit agency? _____

3. By whom are you accredited? _____

4. Are your aides certified or licensed? _____

5. What training do your aides complete in order to get that credential? _____
   _____

6. What special training do aides who work with confused or demented patients receive? _____
   _____

7. What other healthcare professionals do you have on your staff? _____
   _____

8. What supervision do you provide for aides in our home? (You should expect a registered nurse to accompany the aide on the first official day of work and visits by the nurse or other licensed or certified healthcare professionals at regular intervals, perhaps every month or six weeks.) _____
   _____

Finances

9. What are your hourly fees for service? _____
   Does this include: transportation? _____ supervisory visits by other agency personnel (such as the nurse or social worker)? _____
   If not, what are those charges? _____

10. Do you also have a sliding scale fee? _____. Are you managing any special programs or grants under which we could qualify for financial assistance? _____

11. What are the payment arrangements; that is, are we billed weekly, monthly? Do we receive an itemized bill? _____

12. What are your billing arrangements if I should have to keep the aide beyond our previously agreed-upon time (e.g., if I am late from an appointment)? Is it based upon overtime; time-and-a-half; a portion or all of the next hour? _____

Business Arrangements

13. If we should decide to use your agency, is there a contract involved? _____

14. These are the things I need help with. (Have your list handy.) Can you provide these services? ___

15. Is there a waiting list, or can I get someone right away? _____

16. May we have an interview with the aide before hiring her? _____
    (Consider going with another agency if this is not standard practice.)
    How do we arrange this? _____

17. Will you guarantee service if the aide must cancel (for the day, for the whole week, or for two weeks)?
    _____

18. How much notice can we expect if the aide must cancel? _____

19. My relative has always had trouble dealing with certain ethnic or cultural types. We do not necessarily agree with these prejudices, but there is no use trying to change him now. We feel he would be most cooperative with (specify) _____ type of person. Can you help us with that?
_____

20. If for some reason I don't feel comfortable with the person you send, may I request someone else?
_____

21. If the aide is here during a mealtime, will I be expected to provide or will she bring lunch? _____

22. Please send me some literature or a brochure about your agency. Could you also send a copy of any forms that I would have to fill out and a copy of your contract (if there is one)? _____

Your Second Phone Call

My name is _____. I spoke to you over the phone the other day, and I've received your literature. I'd like to arrange for an interview with an aide to help me with some home care. (At this point, list your home care needs again, and be specific about the type of person you are looking for if this is an important issue. See question 19 under Business Arrangements.)

Interviewing The Aide

1. *Observe:* If she is wearing a uniform, is it neat? Clean? _____

    Does her manner seem calm? Poised? _____

    Does she have a pleasant voice? (Remember how important tone of voice is when working with an Alzheimer's person.) _____

Ask the Aide:
2. How long have you been with the agency? _____

3. Tell me a little bit about yourself. How did you happen to get into this type of work? _____
_____

4. What has been your experience with other patients with Alzheimer's disease? _____
_____

5. I need help mostly on _____ (day or days) between _____ (name the hours). (Many caregivers need help between 10:00 a.m. and 2:00 p.m. You may need to be flexible about finding someone during these high demand hours at first.)

    Are you available at these times? _____

If you can't come now at those times, would you be willing to save those times for me later when you are free? _____

For now, when are you available? _____

How soon could you begin? _____

6. Will you bring your lunch, or do you plan to eat here? _____

7. If you are going to eat here during mealtimes, do you have any special food restrictions that I should know about? _____

8. I'd like you to meet my (relative with Alzheimer's). (First, spend a few minutes describing your relative, his feelings, and habits, but not, of course, in front of him.) Observe how the home health aide interacts with him.

How To Communicate Once the Service Has Started

A STEP–BY–STEP MANAGEMENT PROCEDURE

1. Describe in detail the caregiving routines and steps you want the aide to perform. If it is bathing, for example, describe when this is usually done, what methods you have found that work best, and where you typically have trouble with the task.

2. For any new task, *set out all the items* that are needed and show the aide where they should be put away. (This is much more efficient than telling the aide where they are and hoping she will find them when the time comes.)

3. The first time a new task is introduced, stay with the aide to *tell how and when to assist*. The second day you should feel comfortable enough to be in the general vicinity. By the third day you should not feel uncomfortable leaving the house altogether. You will want to find a good balance between leaving even an experienced aide with too much to find out about the situation and hovering to the point of distraction.

   (Experience has shown that, in this new situation, male caregivers tend to stay around but rarely "pitch in." They may be more willing to turn the entire job over to the aide right from the beginning. On the other hand, women may be inclined to want to do the job entirely, finding it difficult to hold back and just instruct and assist.)

OTHER HELPFUL SUGGESTIONS

1. Write out a routine of how the relative spends his day. For example:
    - 9:00   Gets up, washes
    - 10:00 Has breakfast
    - 11:00 Gets dressed, helps feed the dog, etc.

2. Write out a schedule of routines for the week, if there is one:
   Monday: We usually go food shopping
   Tuesday: His granddaughter often stops by
   Wednesday: We try to go for a walk

3. Make a habit of describing to the aide how things went for your relative during the previous night. Relate any major events or behaviors that are out of the ordinary: a cold, a visit to the dentist, a death in the family, an increase in anxiety reactions or withdrawal, etc.

4. Review with the aide the worksheets on sensory deficits and medical conditions that you have filled out in this book. Keep the book handy for her ready reference. She may have valuable information to add.

5. Give the aide (again in writing) a list of the places you are going and approximate times you will be there whenever you leave the house. Leave a phone number where you can be reached and, if possible, the time you will be there. If you are going to be late, call and let her know.

6. Leave a list of where certain things are kept, especially if these are items which you must hide from your relative.

YOUR PERSONAL RELATIONSHIP WITH THE AIDE

1. A good aide will be sensitive to the family structure and attempt to move into your world smoothly. She is available not only for help and companionship for your loved one but also to offer encouragement and support to you. She can also be a valuable resource in showing you how to cope with some tasks you have not been able to figure out yourself. You will gain much by seeing her in the light of all her positive assets and observing how she has been trained to care for persons with Alzheimer's.

2. Discuss any difficulties that arise between the aide and your relative out of the hearing and sight of your relative.

3. If complaints arise from either the aide or your relative about how things are going, have several options for evaluating the problem and finding solutions:

    Do not jump to conclusions. Listen, separately, to the story from both sides.

    Can you find a third party who was in the house at the same time? Perhaps they can give you a view you have not already heard.

    If necessary, ask the aide if you and she can talk together to her supervisor about the problem. Do this in the spirit of finding a solution together so that she won't feel you doubt her or are trying to get her into trouble.

    If you want to take the matter up with the supervisor without the aide's presence, make an appointment with that supervisor in person if at all possible. This gives you a chance to cool down and allows the two of you to discuss the matter in private. It also avoids the risk of having your relative overhear your concerns as you talk over the phone.

GETTING THROUGH: COMMUNICATING WITH A NURSING HOME ADMINISTRATOR

Arriving at a decision to place your relative in a nursing home is neither a quick nor an easy process. However, much of the pain and worry can be reduced by carefully obtaining and comparing information about several nursing homes. Knowing what to ask increases your chances of getting the most useful information, too.

Take time to arrange a tour of the facilities and a personal interview with administrators of each of the homes you are considering. The following questions can be used as a guideline.

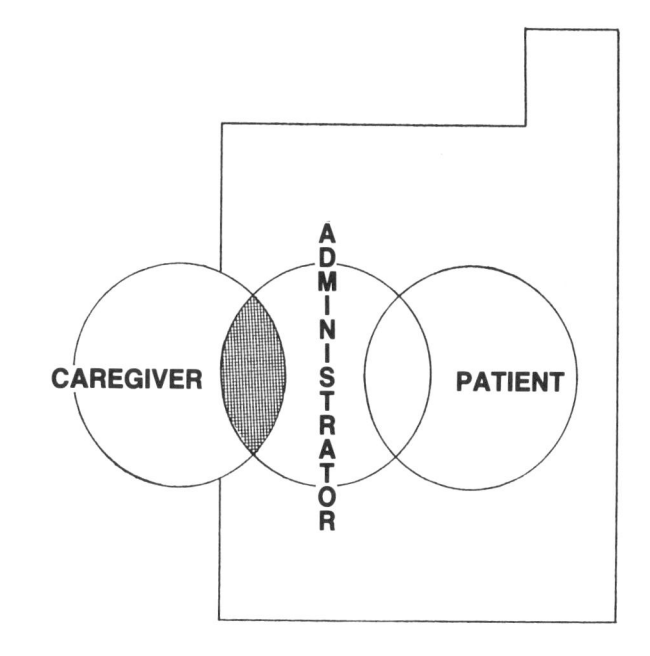

Initial Information

(Over the telephone, a few weeks in advance)

1. We are looking for nursing home placement for my father. Do you accept Alzheimer's patients?

2. Does (or will) your home have beds available for the level of care that has been assigned to my relative? (A level-of-care rating has been assigned by your physician and signifies the amount of skilled nursing time which must be spent with a resident.)

3. Does your home accept the funding sources that we intend to use? (Specify these.)

4. Would you please send us:

    a description of and any brochures about your facility?

    a packet of all the forms that we would have to fill out, including all financial forms?

5. I would like to make an appointment with you to ask some more questions. (If you are already familiar with the home, request an hour; if you have never been there, ask for an hour and a half at least.)

Before each interview, go through this list and circle any questions which have not been clearly explained in the brochures you received. During the appointment, you will find it easier to remember what has been discussed if you ask questions by topic. Take notes too; no one should be offended.

COMMUNICATING WITH THE ADMINISTRATOR

1. Is the home currently licensed by the state? (This license should be displayed prominently in the administrator's office and the current year should be easy to see.)

2. Does the administrator also have a current license from the state? _____

3. Does the home meet or exceed state fire regulations? Can you show me your sprinkler systems and fire doors? What are your evacuation procedures in case of fire? _____

Note: If licensure and safety questions cannot be answered to your satisfaction, it is recommended that this home not be used.

Other questions of great importance are those of accreditation and/or review by peer committees:

1. Is the home accredited by the Long-Term Care Council of the Joint Commission on Accreditation of Hospitals (JCAH?) _____

2. Does the home have a current certificate of review from the state health care or nursing home association's peer review committee? _____

3. Has the home a current certificate to show that it has met standards for other safety and medical criteria? _____

Financial/Medical

1. Go over any points you did not understand about the forms that were sent to you.
   _____
   _____
   _____
   _____

2. Is there an admission fee? A deposit? _____
   How much? _____
   How far in advance must this be paid? _____
   Does this fee apply to the first month's charges? _____

3. Do you accept Medicare and Medicaid patients? _____

   How long is your waiting list for Medicaid beds?
   _____

   (If a private institution:) How many years of private-pay care is required before Medicaid can be initiated?
   _____

4. What is your basic monthly fee? _____
   What does that amount to on a yearly basis? _____
   Does that include the "house" physician's routine checkups? _____

If not, what is the fee? _____
Does that include a dentist's routine checkups? _____
If not, what is the fee? _____

5. What are the fees if we wish the services of the professional barber or hairdresser?
   _____
   An audiologist? _____
   An occupational therapist? _____
   A speech-language pathologist? _____
   A physical therapist? _____
   What procedures are necessary to obtain these services?
   _____
   How will extra services be billed? _____
   By whom, and how often? _____
   Will I receive an itemized account? _____
   Are these professionals only "on call" or are there regularly set times when they can be reached at the facility? _____
   Should my relative require it, is 24-hour nursing care available? _____
   At what cost? _____
   How is it obtained? _____
   What about costs and procedures for obtaining laundry services, extra nursing supplies (such as diaper pads), or medications? _____
   _____

6. If we need to arrange for outside appointments (for instance, a required medical service):
   Who arranges the transportation? _____
   Who pays for the transportation? _____
   What is the fee? _____
   _____

7. Should I arrange to have our physician see my relative, or do you have a staff physician who makes regular calls? _____
   _____
   How often? _____
   What is the best way to keep in touch with the house physician? _____
   _____
   What if I prefer for our physician to continue to see my relative? _____
   _____
   Is there a professional courtesy I should be aware of? _____
   _____

8. What is your policy on heroic measures for a terminally ill patient? _____
   _____
   Will the nursing home follow the family's wishes in this matter? _____

9. Suppose there are some items in the contract that I could not agree with. Are any portions of the contract negotiable? (Most are not.) _____

Resident Care

1. Are confused patients grouped together on the same floor, ward, or wing? _____

    May we visit this area? _____

    How do you handle wandering? With restraints? Exit door alarms? Plastic flaps? (The latter is preferable because alarms may be frightening.)

    _____

2. How do you handle incontinence? _____

    Do you take the patient to the toilet every two hours or at regular intervals?

    _____

3. Who provides consultation, training, or supervision for patients who develop swallowing problems? (Ideally, this is a team approach by a speech-language pathologist, an occupational therapist, and/or a dietician.)

    Can you describe what treatment or dietary steps are taken before a decision is made to begin tube feeding? _____

    (This question, like those about wandering, incontinence, and special grouping, may seem very technical, but it is important that you be perceived by the administration as a knowledgeable healthcare consumer who wants to learn and be informed.)

Quality of Life and Recreation

1. Do you have an orientation board for the patients? _____
    (This is a large bulletin board or calendar that shows such things as the date, weather, special events, activities, birthdays, and day's menus.)

2. What activities do you have specifically for the more confused or demented residents? _____

    Is music or music therapy a frequent part of your routine? _____
    What about pets and pet therapy? _____

    Do you have supervised daily exercise? _____

3. Is there a structured schedule? _____
    Do you provide a weekly (or monthly) calendar? If I know about a special event ahead of time, may I join in? _____

4. How do you provide for religious or other dietary restrictions? _____

   How frequently do you receive visits from clergy of our faith? (Or is this only by special request to our own minister?) _____

   Which religious services are held here, and when? _____

5. Do you have any restrictions on personal possessions we should know about? _____

Staff Credentials and Training

1. What is the ratio of nursing staff to patients? Of aides to patients? _____
   What is your rate of staff turnover? (A good clue to staff satisfaction, this rate should be no higher than 40-50% per year.) _____

   About how many hours each year does the staff who works directly with the demented or confused patients receive specific training in dementia and geriatric care? _____
   Who provides the training? _____

Your Role

1. Are any of the following groups affiliated with your nursing home? How do I contact:
   An Alzheimer's support group? _____
   An education or advocacy group? _____
   A relatives' advisory group? _____

2. What are your suggestions for my family's role in our relative's care? _____

A FINAL WORD

No single book can be all things to all people. Each victim is at a different stage of this sad disease called Alzheimer's. Each family is at a different phase of acceptance. Each reader comes with a different set of motivations. Whether you are primary caregiver, friend, healthcare worker, or just a casual acquaintance, we hope the ideas contained in this book have helped you in some way. If so, then our goal of getting through to you will have been met.

Perhaps now you can see your loved one's faltering attempts at communication in a more positive light and are able to respond with new understanding and thoughtfulness. Maybe you have become more sensitive to your own emotions and attitudes which flavor and color your every communicative act.

You may have discovered you are at your creative best as you involve yourself in developing an environment that is more supportive of the human need to communicate. We hope you have acquired both courage and skill in speaking with unfamiliar persons about uncomfortable topics. We hope too you have learned that asking provocative questions may be the best way to obtain reliable and useful information.

In every life and in every experience, nothing is as rewarding as getting through to another person. So much is at stake between two human beings and between past and future generations. "Getting through" is a *process* – a process in which one continually learns, eternally becomes. Wherever you are on your journey, Godspeed.

APPENDIX

Healthcare Professionals: Consumer Information

Where to Get More Information

APPENDIX A

HEALTHCARE PROFESSIONALS: CONSUMER INFORMATION

HEALTHCARE PROVIDER	EDUCATIONAL CREDENTIALS	WHERE TO FIND	INFORMATION YOU NEED TO BRING	WHAT THEY CAN HELP YOU WITH
Audiologist Jane Doe, M.A., CCC-A	**Minimum Requirements** Master's Degree plus Certificate of Clinical Competence (CCC) from American Speech-Language-Hearing Association Licensure (in most states)	**In Yellow Pages under** Audiology **Types of Settings** Private Practice Hospitals Clinics Rehabilitation Centers Nursing Homes University Clinics Some Physicians' or Dentists' Offices **Address of National Office** American Speech-Language-Hearing Association 10801 Rockville Pike Rockville, MD 20852 **National Office Phone Number** 1-301-897-5700 or for consumer information: 1-800-638-8255	Past medical history including: Ear infections Head injury Allergies Medications Recreational history (such as water sports: swimming, diving, or scuba diving) History of prolonged noise exposure: military, occupational, or recreational Records from any previous audiological tests Bring hearing aid if owns one, whether it is used or not	Detection/diagnosis of hearing loss Hearing aid evaluation and fitting Counseling regarding wearing and adjusting to hearing aid or adjustment to hearing impairment Information about • assistive listening devices • speech (lip) reading • aural rehabilitation

HEALTHCARE PROFESSIONALS: CONSUMER INFORMATION

HEALTHCARE PROVIDER	EDUCATIONAL CREDENTIALS	WHERE TO FIND	INFORMATION YOU NEED TO BRING	WHAT THEY CAN HELP YOU WITH
Clinical Nutritionist or **Registered Dietician** Jane Doe, R.D.	**Minimum Requirements** Bachelor's Degree plus National certification required in order to practice Licensure required in some states	**In Yellow Pages under** Nutritionists **Types of Settings** Hospitals Nursing Homes Business and Industry Private Practice University Settings Home Health Care **Address of National Office** American Dietetic Association 430 North Michigan Avenue Chicago, IL 60611 **National Office Phone Number** 1-800-621-6469	Patient's medical and physical history, specifically: Medications Dental status Any chewing or swallowing problems Food allergies and dietary restrictions Significant weight gain or loss over recent months Assistance needed during mealtimes Patient's ability to recall if meals or medications have been (or must be) taken Any other specific concerns (e.g., chronic constipation)	Provide information counseling and therapy including Evaluate client's nutritional needs and make appropriate recommendations to client and to other medical team members Monitor correct diet Develop and assist with hospital, nursing home, and community programs

HEALTHCARE PROFESSIONALS: CONSUMER INFORMATION

HEALTHCARE PROVIDER	EDUCATIONAL CREDENTIALS	WHERE TO FIND	INFORMATION YOU NEED TO BRING	WHAT THEY CAN HELP YOU WITH
Homemaker/Home Health Aide Jane Doe	**Minimum Requirements** According to individual state requirements aides must have a certain number of specialized hours in training before their services are reimbursable by Medicare or Medicaid Aides in nonprofit agencies may also be accredited member of that state's Home Care Council The Agency is required to hold certification and/or licensure in order for their services to be reimbursed by Medicare or Medicaid. Such credentials assure better quality of service even when reimbursement is not the issue	**In Yellow Pages under** Home Health Services Community Services, under "Health" **Types of Settings** Public and private nonprofit and for-profit agencies **Address of National Office** National Home Caring Council 235 Park Avenue South New York, NY 10003 **National Office Phone Number** 1-212-674-4990	Patient's medical history and medications Patient's physician's name and phone Information about Medicare or Medicaid benefits Description of patient's daily routine/schedule Need for special services of practical or registered nurse Hours and days of services needed List of services needed: BE AS SPECIFIC AS POSSIBLE	Offer companionship and socialization Personal care of patient (bath, skin care, shampoo, etc.) Essential errands (going to grocery store, pharmacy, laundromat, etc.) Prepare meals, including special diets Assist with medications Assist with therapy programs Perform light household chores Care for children when mother is ill

HEALTHCARE PROFESSIONALS: CONSUMER INFORMATION

HEALTHCARE PROVIDER	EDUCATIONAL CREDENTIALS	WHERE TO FIND	INFORMATION YOU NEED TO BRING	WHAT THEY CAN HELP YOU WITH
Nurse Clinician Jane Doe, M.S.M., R.N. or: M.S.N., R.N.C* *(If certified by national certification boards)	**Minimum Requirements** Master's Degree in speciality area (oncology, geriatrics, etc.) *Certification must be updated at specified intervals, from two to five years	**In Yellow Pages under** Not applicable/see below **Types of Settings** Healthcare Organizations, such as: Day Hospital Diagnostic Clinic Resource Center Clinics Research Center Hospitals Some Nursing Homes **Address of National Office** American Nurses Association 2420 Pershing Road Kansas City, MO 64108 **National Office Phone Number** 1-800-821-5834	Information regarding Medications (bring in list or actual bottles) Eating habits Grooming Hygiene Ability to do household chores Life changes in past two years Sleeping patterns Legal problems Housing problems Information regarding health status, employment, stress, and general level of functioning of primary caregiver	Determine level of functioning of patient and caregiver Determine mental status of patient Identify possible medical conditions that could be complicating health status Develop an overall management plan in consultation with physician(s) Develop a management plan in conjunction with family based on their needs and resources Provide education and answers related to dementia, aging, and Alzheimer's Counseling regarding nutrition and safety Assistance with future planning Assistance in filling out forms
Gerontological Nurse Jane Doe, B.S.N., R.N.C.*	**Minimum Requirements** Bachelor's Degree			

HEALTHCARE PROFESSIONALS: CONSUMER INFORMATION

HEALTHCARE PROVIDER	EDUCATIONAL CREDENTIALS	WHERE TO FIND	INFORMATION YOU NEED TO BRING	WHAT THEY CAN HELP YOU WITH
Occupational Therapist Jane Doe, O.T.R.	**Minimum Requirements** Bachelor's Degree Licensure required in some states	**In Yellow Pages under** Occupational Therapist **Types of Settings** Adult Day Care Settings Acute Care Hospitals Rehabilitation Hospitals Outpatient Clinics Health/Home Care Agencies University Clinics Nursing Homes **Address of National Office** American Occupational Therapy Association, Inc. 1383 Piccard Drive Rockville, MD 20850 **National Office Phone Number** 1-301-948-9626	Prescription from physician Pertinent medical information Description of physical set-up of home: steps, bathroom access Ability to care for self: dressing, feeding, daily hygiene	Assist patient and family with ways to achieve best functioning in daily activities and to help maintain patient's self-care ability as long as possible Explore with family new approaches to work with patient Provide general conditioning exercises for patient Provide education for family relative to expectations and course of difficulties. Foster awareness of present capabilities

HEALTHCARE PROFESSIONALS: CONSUMER INFORMATION

HEALTHCARE PROVIDER	EDUCATIONAL CREDENTIALS	WHERE TO FIND	INFORMATION YOU NEED TO BRING	WHAT THEY CAN HELP YOU WITH
Patient Activities Coordinator (or Recreational Therapist, Music Therapist, Art Therapist Jane Doe, C.T.R.S. or Jane Doe, R.M.T. or Jane Doe, A.T.R.	**Minimum Requirements** Bachelor's Degree with major in recreation or occupational therapy or related field such as art, music, physical education, group work, or sociology or: Associate Degree in Recreation *plus* two years' experience in recreational therapy for the aged, handicapped, or developmentally delayed National Certification, laws pending	**In Yellow Pages under** Contact individual facilities **Types of Settings** Adult Day Care Centers Senior Citizen Centers Rehabilitation Centers Mental Health Facilities Psychiatric Facilities Nursing Homes **Address of National Office** National Association of Activity Professionals P.O. Box 274 Park Ridge, IL 60068 **National Office Phone Number** 1-312-692-2564	In general: Knowledge of the individual's former life style, including interests, job, hobbies, educational level, and religious preference In addition: In nursing homes must have a physician's orders (speak to the floor nurses and they will relay the request to the doctor or you can contact the doctor directly)	Assess patient's physical condition (alertness, confusion, orientation), special needs or diets, and psychosocial functioning Focus on activities that challenge, stimulate, and encourage the person to meet their • spiritual • physical • psychosocial • intellectual needs Individual, small group, or large group setting Provide informal instruction to family members for doing same activities with patient; serves as resource for other meaningful activities

HEALTHCARE PROFESSIONALS: CONSUMER INFORMATION

HEALTHCARE PROVIDER	EDUCATIONAL CREDENTIALS	WHERE TO FIND	INFORMATION YOU NEED TO BRING	WHAT THEY CAN HELP YOU WITH
Physical Therapist John Doe, R.P.T. or L.P.T. or P.T.	**Minimum Requirements** Bachelor's Degree plus Must be approved by Americal Physical Therapy Association Also: Current State Licensure	**In Yellow Pages under** Physical Therapists Physical Therapy Rehabiliation Services **Types of Settings** Hospitals Nursing Homes Rehabilitation Centers Visiting Nurses Agencies Private Practice **Address of National Office** American Physical Therapy Association 1111 North Fairfax Street Alexandria, VA 22314 **National Office Phone Number** 703-684-2782	Physician's prescription for therapy (including pertinent diagnoses)	Musculoskeletal and neurological problems which result in loss of movement, strength, walking ability, etc. *Examples:* Arthritis Stroke/Head injury Pinched nerve Nerve damage Amputation Burns Spinal injuries Cancer General weakness and deconditioning

HEALTHCARE PROFESSIONALS: CONSUMER INFORMATION

HEALTHCARE PROVIDER	EDUCATIONAL CREDENTIALS	WHERE TO FIND	INFORMATION YOU NEED TO BRING	WHAT THEY CAN HELP YOU WITH
Social Worker Jane Doe, M.S.W. or John Doe, A.C.S.W.*	**Minimum Requirements** Master's Degree Academy of Certified Social Workers* *(Requires special study, a national examination, and time spent in internship) Licensure also required in some states	**In Yellow Pages under** Social Work Mental Health Counseling Agencies Family Therapy Social Service Agencies **Types of Settings** Hospitals and Clinics Mental Health Agencies Family Service Agencies Home Health Agencies Social Service Agencies Nursing Homes Private Practice **Address of National Office** National Association of Social Workers 7981 Eastern Avenue Silver Spring, MD 20910 **National Office Phone Number** Not Applicable (Not in service for consumer information)	If you need information about financial resources, have knowledge or documents about current income source and the date first pay was received If you need information about insurance, bring in current policy, if any	Counseling regarding Personal, mental, family problems Financial concerns Referral to appropriate community resources, agencies, or other professionals who might be helpful Possible extended care options for the elderly disabled (e.g., nursing home placement, skilled, or 24-hour nursing care, etc.) Referral to community support groups Assistance in filling out forms

HEALTHCARE PROFESSIONALS: CONSUMER INFORMATION

HEALTHCARE PROVIDER	EDUCATIONAL CREDENTIALS	WHERE TO FIND	INFORMATION YOU NEED TO BRING	WHAT THEY CAN HELP YOU WITH
Speech-Language Pathologist Jane Doe, M.A., CCC-SLP	**Minimum Requirements** Master's Degree Certificate of Clinical Competence (CCC) Licensure (in most states)	**In Yellow Pages under** Speech-Language Pathologist **Types of Settings** Private Practice Hospitals Rehabilitation Centers University Clinics Home Health Care Nursing Homes **Address of National Office** American Speech-Language-Hearing Association 10801 Rockville Pike Rockville, MD 20852 **National Office Phone Number** 1-301-897-5700 or for consumer information: 1-800-638-8255	Any information regarding previous speech, language, or hearing evaluation or treatment Reports of medical status of patient, especially previous stroke, head trauma, or degenerative disease Any medications Any chewing or swallowing difficulties Reports of dental and visual tests Description of patient's current behavior, especially communication skills and important communication situations	Assessing level of language comprehension and use Facilitating maximum use of available language Counseling on how best to interact with patient Aiding adjustment and use of hearing aid Treatment of swallowing disorders (dysphagia)

HEALTHCARE PROFESSIONALS: CONSUMER INFORMATION

HEALTHCARE PROVIDER	EDUCATIONAL CREDENTIALS	WHERE TO FIND	INFORMATION YOU NEED TO BRING	WHAT THEY CAN HELP YOU WITH
Visiting Nurse Jane Doe, R.N.	**Minimum requirement** Associate Degree (2 years) (3 or 4 year degree required for some duties and positions) For reimbursement for Medicare or Medicaid patients, the Visiting Nurse Home Care Agency *itself* must also have licensure and/or certification through the individual state's Department of Health May also be accredited by National League for Nursing Look for Agency's participation in the Chronic Care Program for the Elderly and Disabled (CCPED)	**In Yellow Pages under** Nurses Home Health Physical Therapy In white pages: Visiting Nurses Also: Senior Citizens Silver Pages **Types of Settings** Agency Offices Also provide services in home settings, clinics, health departments, nursing homes, or boarding homes **Address of National Office** National Association for Home Care 519 "C" Street, NE Stanton Park, Washington, DC 20002 **National Office Phone Number** 1-202-547-7424	For initial visit: Name, address, phone number, physician's name For follow-up visits: Medical prescription from physician, including Plan of treatment Medications Diagnosis Prognosis History of physical condition and what physician has in mind for home care (Note: for Medicare or Blue Cross insurance, physician must also signify that patient is truly homebound. May not be necessary for other companies)	Arranging for: Skilled nursing Physical therapy Occupational therapy Speech-language pathology Social services Consultations Nutritionist Home health aides Some agencies also employ a Clinical Nurse Specialist whose speciality is in gerontology, rehabilitation, oncology, etc. (See page 77 of this Appendix) Help with filling out forms Other support services such as bath services may be available

APPENDIX B

WHERE TO GET MORE INFORMATION

ALZHEIMER'S DISEASE AND RELATED DISORDERS ASSOCIATION (ADRDA)
70 East Lake Street
Chicago, IL 60601
1-312-853-3060

AMERICAN SPEECH-LANGUAGE-HEARING ASSOCIATION (ASHA)
10801 Rockville Pike
Rockville, MD 20852
1-800-638-8255

MEDIC ALERT FOUNDATION INTERNATIONAL
Turlock, CA 95381
1-800-344-3226

REFERENCES

Bayles, K.A. and Kaszniak, A.W. *Communication and cognition in normal aging and dementia.* Boston: Little, Brown, 1987.

Bayles, K.A. Language and dementia. In A.L. Holland (ed.) *Language disorders in adults: Recent advances.* San Diego: College-Hill, 1984.

Blazer, D. and Williams, C.D. Epidemiology of dysphoria and depression in an elderly population. *American Journal of Psychiatry,* 1980, *137,* 439-444.

Cook, J. In consultation with M.J. Santo Pietro and P. Schneider. Yes, I can hear you. *Fifty Plus.* August 1979.

Cross, P.S. and Gurland, B.J. *The epidemoiology of dementing disorders.* A report on work performed by and submitted to the United States Congress, Office of Technology Assessment. New York: Columbia University Center for Geriatrics, Gerontology, and Long-Term Care, 1985.

Griffith, J. and Strandberg, T. *A guide to nursing home living.* Charleston, IL: Generations, 1982.

Halpern Audiotapes. Belmont, CA: Halpern Sounds, 1979.

Holland, L.J. *Reality oriented communication training for senile dementia patients.* Doctoral dissertation, University of Utah. Ann Arbor: University Microfilms, 1984.

Hill, R.H. Demography and characteristics of the communication disordered elderly. *Seminars in Speech Language Hearing,* 1981, *2,* 137-148.

Lubinski, R. (ed.) *Dementia and communication.* Philadelphia: B.C. Decker, 1991.

Lubinski, R.; Morrison, E.B.; and Rigrodsky, S. Perception of spoken communication by elderly chronically ill patients in an institutional setting. *Journal of Speech and Hearing Disorders,* 1981, *46,* 405-412.

Mace, N.L. and Rabins, P.V. *The 36-hour day: A family guide to caring for persons with Alzheimer's disease, related dementing illnesses, and memory loss in late life.* Baltimore/London: Johns Hopkins, 1982.

Rowe, J. and Besdine, R. *Health and disease in old age.* Boston: Little, Brown, 1982.

Shadden, B. *Communication behavior and aging: A sourcebook for clinicians.* Baltimore: Williams and Wilkins, 1988.

Santo Pietro, M.J.; DeCotiis, E.; McCarthy, J.M.; and Ostuni, E. *Conversation in Alzheimer's disease: Implications of semantic and pragmatic breakdowns.* Paper presented at the annual meeting of the American Speech-Language-Hearing Association, Seattle, WA, November 17, 1990.

Santo Pietro, M.J. and Goldfarb, R. Characteristic patterns of word association responses in institutionalized elderly with and without senile dementia. *Brain and Language,* 1984, *26,* 230-243.

Tanner, F. and Shaw, S. *Caring: A family guide to managing the Alzheimer's patient at home.* New York: New York City Alzheimer's Resource Center, 1985.

Ulatowska, H.K. *The aging brain: Communication in the elderly.* San Diego: College-Hill, 1985.

Windham Hill Tapes. *Water's path.* Hollywood, CA: Paramount Home Video, 1984.

ABOUT THE AUTHORS

Elizabeth Ostuni is a Speech-Language Pathologist and Director, Accent on Communication, Sparta, New Jersey. She was formerly Director of Speech-Language Pathology and Audiology Services and Coordinator, Alzheimer's Functional Assessment Team, Dover General Hospital, Dover, New Jersey. President of the New Jersey Speech-Language-Hearing Association 1991-1992, she is also the author of *Sound Investments*.

Mary Jo Santo Pietro is Professor of Speech-Language Pathology and Associate Director of the Speech and Hearing Center at Herbert H. Lehman College, City University of New York. She conducts research in communication disorders in the elderly and has published numerous articles in scientific journals. She is a Fellow of the American Speech-Language-Hearing Association and formerly Vice President of Governmental Affairs for the New Jersey Speech-Language-Hearing Association.